THINGS I'VE LEARNED FROM DYING:
A BOOK ABOUT LIFE

ALSO BY DAVID R. DOW

The Autobiography of an Execution

THINGS I'VE LEARNED FROM DYING

A Book about Life

DAVID R. DOW

TWELVE

Grand Central Press

New York Boston

Pablo Neruda, excerpt from "No me lo pidan", CANCIÓN DE GESTA © Fundación Pablo Neruda, 2013

Twelve
Hachette Book Group
237 Park Avenue
New York, NY 10017
www.HachetteBookGroup.com

Book design by Carin Dow
Printed in the United States of America

RRD-C

First Edition: January 2014

10 9 8 7 6 5 4 3 2 1

Twelve is an imprint of Grand Central Publishing.
The Twelve name and logo are trademarks of Hachette Book Group, Inc.

The Hachette Speakers Bureau provides a wide range of authors for speaking events. To find out more, go to www.hachettespeakersbureau.com or call (866) 376-6591.

The publisher is not responsible for websites (or their content) that are not owned by the publisher.

Library of Congress Cataloging-in-Publication Data has been applied for.

ISBN (hardcover): 978-1-455-57524-4

For Katya and Lincoln,
my pillars

I could write a book about what I don't know.

—Ryan Bingham, "I Don't Know"

Every life is different, but every death is the same. We live with others. We die alone. And what is important to this story is that the moment we die is not the same as the moment we are perceived as dead. Our lives end before others notice, and the time that spans that distance is the inverse of the grief your loved ones will suffer when you leave them behind.

A week after one of my clients was executed, I was talking to a room full of lawyers at the state bar convention in Fort Worth. I described his final day, how he showered and shaved then put on clean clothes and took a ninety-minute van ride from death row in Livingston to the Walls Unit in Huntsville, where he was executed at thirteen minutes past six. I told the lawyers how earlier that day I watched his mother, father, sister, and brother tell him good-bye. One man asked whether they had been able to embrace. I said no, there are no contact visits with death row inmates. Another asked how long he had been on death row. I told her six years and eight months. She said, His family had six years and eight months longer to say good-bye than his victim's family had.

Which is better: to be able to circle the date on a calendar five years from today when your life will end? Or to get flattened by a truck crossing the street and never see it coming? Who had the easier death: Timothy McVeigh, or his victims?

I'm not going to argue with you, no matter what you say. One thing I've learned is that the answer to the question isn't obvious.

BEGINNINGS

The same sequence of days can arrange themselves into a number of different stories.

—Jane Smiley, *A Thousand Acres*

met my future father-in-law at Ruggle's Grille the night Katya graduated from law school. There were six of us. Peter and Irmi wanted to drink champagne to celebrate their daughter's achievement. He asked the waiter to bring us two bottles.

Peter was born in 1938. Hitler had already annexed the Sudetenland. When the Wehrmacht invaded the rest of Czechoslovakia in March 1939, Peter was wearing diapers. But on the night we met, I could not make myself picture him as a year-old toddler crawling shirtless across the floor of his nursery just outside Berlin. He came to the United States as a young adult with a Ph.D. in chemistry from the University of Munich. He had angular Teutonic features, and he spoke with a hard High German accent. I sat there sipping Tattinger, wondering what his father had been doing while my family was fleeing the Nazis, or being gassed by them.

At the age of forty, Peter traded what he loved, being a laboratory scientist, for what he despised, being a manager. I asked him why he did it. He had a wife and two children. He was holding Irmi's hand. He said, *The money, young man. The money.* He showed us pictures of the house he and Irmi were building on the lake, his retirement home. There was a slip for his sailboat and custom-designed slots for his windsurfer and kayaks. Thirty-five years earlier, before the lines of

3

people climbing Mount Everest looked like an ad from L.L. Bean, back in the days when backcountry hikers had to know how to pull their own brisket out of the fire, Peter had trekked across Nepal and Bhutan, giving away his penicillin to kids with dark green snot oozing from their nostrils, and being hailed as an angel when he passed through the same villages on his way back home. I asked him what was so bad about upper management. He said, *You have to fire people.*

My zaide, my grandfather, used to tell me you have two ears and one mouth because you are supposed to listen twice as much as you talk. By that logic, Peter had ten ears. That night he asked me what I was writing and reading; he asked what I liked most about teaching and what I liked least. He asked about my parents and wanted to know what my four younger brothers did for a living. He did not ask about my clients on death row, or why I represent them. He was too decorous to ask so intrusive a question on the night we met.

He did ask about the semester I spent in Israel. I lived in Tel Aviv. I told him about my downstairs neighbors, a young couple so German they were a caricature. Their eyes were sapphire and their hair was blond. Her breakfast was strong coffee, a pretzel, and a cigarette. He wore black socks with his tan open-toed sandals. They insisted on speaking only Hebrew, even when alone. I asked them why. Both their fathers had been Brown Shirts, so they moved to Israel and worked at an orphanage as expiation. I told Peter about them. I said, I think they were nuts.

He said, *I don't think so. Not at all. What they did makes perfect sense to me.*

■ ■ ■

The thirty-two-year-old nurse was filling her tank at two in the morning at a gas station where the lone employee was a middle-age Korean man who sat on a stool in a booth behind bulletproof Plexiglas and wouldn't come out even to pee if anyone was nearby. Four young black men pulled up driving a maroon Ford LTD. One stepped out and said, Gimme the bag, bitch. She didn't even hesitate, but he backhanded her anyway, using the hand that held his gun. The clerk later told police he could hear her jaw crack. She lay on the ground, just conscious enough to register the steel toes in the boots her assailant was wearing when he kicked her in the ribs. She heard him say to the other three men in the car, Let's get the fuck out of here. Her name was Tamira, and she'd never forget his voice, or his face.

It was the beginning of a weeklong bender that ended with murder on a cool fall evening in a white-flight suburb north of Dallas. The same four had parked the LTD at the curb in front of Lucy McClain's Tudor-style home. One stayed with the car, the other three finished their beers, tossed the cans on the manicured lawn, and walked up to the house.

Miss McClain was upstairs in bed, watching the news and knitting. She was eighty-four years old, with rheumy blue eyes and brittle white hair. A copy of *O Magazine* was on the night table, under her reading glasses, next to a smudged glass of lukewarm water she planned to use to wash down her nightly pills.

Demetrius Sanders said to the others, Y'all ready to do this? And he kicked in the door. He was eighteen. Eddie Waterman and his cousin, Harold Johnston, were nineteen. They led the way upstairs. The TV was turned up loud. Miss McClain probably did not hear the intruders until they entered her room. She clutched the knitting tightly in front of her breasts. She was scared, but she was calm. She told them they could have whatever they wanted. Waterman walked over to the night table. He had been a linebacker on his high school football team and had been recruited to play college ball at Oklahoma. He was massive, with short hair and a tattoo that identified his gang. Miss McClain cowered. He picked up a set of car keys.

Johnston pulled a gun from his waistband. Sanders said, What you doin', man?

Johnston looked at Sanders and shrugged. He looked at Miss McClain, then he shot her in the left temple. The bullet exited through her right ear. Waterman jumped back. His left arm was covered with brains and blood. He said, Fuck, man.

Miss McClain was dead. Johnston handed the gun to Waterman. He took it and held it sideways. He fired a shot into her lifeless body. The slug from the 9 mm pistol entered Miss McClain's left mandible, pierced her tongue, and exited through the bottom of her mouth. Waterman handed back the gun to Johnston. He said, That's how you smoke a bitch.

■ ■ ■

ix months before his retirement party Peter felt a lump two centimeters below the left edge of his right scapula. He thought it was a persistent mosquito bite, but he asked Irmi to feel it anyway. She did, and she became alarmed. She urged him to see his doctor.

He did not heed her advice. For three months Peter held to his belief it was a bite. Irmi asked him again to have an expert look. He said he would, but for another two months, he did not. He finally went to his own doctor, a Hopkins graduate who practiced medicine in a strip mall office past the Woodlands off I-45. He was crammed between a Subway and a manicurist, and in the waiting room you could smell bread baking and hear chatter in a language that might have been Thai. The biggest cancer center in the world was forty miles south.

Katya and Irmi implored him to see an oncologist at M.D. Anderson, but he delayed for two weeks longer. He said, *I cannot do that. It would be insulting to the young man who has taken good care of me for two years.* He finally agreed to let the doctor cut it out, and even when his doctor urged him to see someone else, Peter did not.

Irmi finally made the appointment for him anyway. He went only because it would have been rude to cancel. He went back because he was impressed. The doctor said, It's unusual. I wish you had come to see me sooner. Hearing that, Irmi felt fear, not satisfaction.

He was fifty-eight years old. His plan to spend the next year hiking and windsurfing and kayaking was imperiled by the fact he might not be alive for another year. His loyalty and denial were complicit in creating his predicament. Later he would know that.

A B C D is the dermatologist's mnemonic for melanoma: A for asymmetry, B for border irregularity, C for color variation, D for diameter. Answer yes to any question and what looks like an ordinary mole is a Trojan horse carrying a miserable death. The lump on Peter's back was four for four. It was large and it was ulcerated, two especially bad signs. The only remaining question was whether the cancer was already in his bloodstream, looking for beachheads in his lungs, liver, and brain. He was a scientist and an intellectual. The one thing he feared was losing his brain.

The doctor told Peter he needed immediate surgery to remove lymph nodes and probably chemotherapy after that. Peter called to tell us from the house on the lake. He was sitting outside so Irmi would not hear the despair in his voice. In the background I could hear waves splashing against the bulkhead. When we got off the phone Katya broke down. She said, I'm not even crying because he has cancer. I can hear it in his voice. He's already given up.

Two days later Peter packed an overnight bag and drove wordlessly to Houston while Irmi sat beside him unable to read. He asked her to please go sleep at our house but she refused. She bought hot tea in the hospital cafeteria and paced the halls waiting for Peter to fall asleep, but every time she opened the door to his room, he looked at her and said, *Not yet*. Nurses walked in every two hours and wrote numbers on charts. At six they wheeled him into pre-op, and for the first time in a week he thawed. He let Irmi kiss him on the cheek. He held her hand in both of his, then held it to his mouth and said he loved her. She watched him recede around the corner, then went back to the room to wait. Katya and I arrived minutes before the surgeon. He came in and said everything went well. He had removed three nodes with minimal damage to surrounding tissue. If he told us his name, I missed it. He had all the charm of a traffic cop. Irmi started to ask him how to care for the wounds but he cut her off, said the nurse would answer any questions, and was gone half a minute after he'd arrived.

Peter went home the next day. The oncologist reminded him the first round of chemo would start in two weeks and told him to eat as much as he could between now and then. Peter didn't tell him he might not be back. He wasn't telling anyone yet that he wasn't committed to the plan.

Melanoma staging uses three variables: T, N, and M. T refers to tumor size, the thinner the better; N stands for lymph nodes; and M is short for metastasis to other organs. Each of the three variables also has subvariables. For example, if a tumor is relatively thin (less than 1 mm), the staging calculation further relies on the tumor's mitotic rate, which is an indication of how quickly the cancer cells are dividing (i.e., replicating).

Peter's tumor was T4b-N2b-Mx. The tumor (T) was thicker than 4 mm (it was 4.15 mm) and ulcerated. There was macroscopic spread to at least two lymph nodes (N). The M value was unknown because the doctors were unsure whether there were tumors in other organs. If there were, his tumor was stage IV. If not, his tumor was stage IIIc, just a hair's breadth better than the worst there is.

■　■　■

Katya and Irmi were inside unpacking boxes of shark cartilage and garlic capsules they'd ordered from a shaman online. Peter and I were sitting outside on the deck, looking out at the lake. After he read me the pathology report he took off his glasses and rubbed his eyes. He said, *One drawback of being a scientist is I am aware it is hopeless. If I elect to do nothing further, Irmi and I can drive out west. We can hike and camp and live. I can die on a mountain. If we remain here, I will die in diapers in an air-conditioned room.*

Winona came running around the side of the house. There were two tall pines, four feet apart. Winona ran between them, carrying a five-foot limb, and slammed into an invisible wall. She took three steps back, turned ninety degrees, and stepped through the trees. Peter said, *That dog is smarter than me.* He took the branch from Winona and slung it into the lake. She dived in after it.

I said, If you run away, this is what you'll miss.

He threw the stick three more times then said, *Enough.* Winona lay down between us, her head resting on Peter's bare foot. He asked what was going on with me. I told him I had been appointed by a federal judge to represent a new client. He said, *Two men without a chance drifting to their fates.*

I said, Maybe my client, but not you. You have options, you know.

You're not a leaf in the breeze. The chemo might work. There are other therapies. You don't know enough to give up.

And I thought to myself, *And your acting like your life is already over is driving your wife and daughter crazy.*

He said, *The power of will can be overstated. My tumor is greater than four millimeters in thickness and ulcerated. It's probably spread. The five-year survival rate for people with this tumor is less than 50 percent. You think the people who lose the coin flip don't want to live as much as the ones who win?*

Among death penalty lawyers, inmates who want to surrender their appeals and march straight to the execution chamber are known as volunteers. Some lawyers think that anyone who volunteers is by definition mentally ill, and they try to thwart their clients' desire to give up. But death row inmates spend twenty-three hours a day in a sixty-square-foot cell with a solid steel door and a slit of translucent plastic for a window. They do not have televisions or computers. They have one hour a day of solitary exercise and three showers per week. Their food comes from vending machines or cans. They get two radio stations. Barely literate, they couldn't occupy their days reading even if they had the patience to do so. At conferences, I am not just being the devil's advocate when I argue volunteers can be rational. I said to Peter, The fact that a good attitude won't save you doesn't mean a bad attitude won't kill you.

He said, *It's the treatment that will kill me. I know how the chemicals work. The methylating agents interfere with the ability of the cancer cells to replicate. They'll drip 200 milligrams of dacarbazine into me for five days. On the first day and on the last, they'll add 3 milligrams of vindesine to the cocktail. In between, I'll take lomustine orally, probably around 100 milligrams, and another 15 milligrams of bicomysin subcutaneously on days one and four. The doctor told me the toxicity level of this mix is acceptable. By that he means acceptable to* him. *From my perspective, it is a week off what remains of my life. Do you know there is not one documented case of a remission using this approach? Even in a best-case scenario, the poison won't cure me. Maybe it gets me another three months. Maybe six. Maybe none, in which case I've traded seven days for nothing.*

He paused and looked back over his shoulder. Through the window we could see Katya and Irmi setting the table. Peter and I were going to grill a leg of lamb. He said, *It does no good to discuss this with Katya. She loves me. It clouds her judgment.*

I said, Love does not cloud her judgment. It gives her perspective. If the only people you're going to talk to are people who don't care about you, you are probably not going to hear anything you're interested in listening to.

He said, *Maybe that is why monks stop talking.*

He scratched Winona behind the ears and rubbed his eyes. He hadn't yet lost his taste for champagne. He took a swallow and waited for me to argue. When I didn't, he said, *Let's go cook the lamb.*

After we put the meat on the grill, he asked, *What did your client do?*

I said, His name is Waterman. He killed somebody.

It's a joke among death penalty lawyers. That's always what they did. I told him about Miss McClain.

Peter said, *And why exactly do you want to save this man?*

I said, I'm not sure yet.

■ ■ ■

atya and I got Winona before we were married. We bought her when she was six weeks old from a breeder in Waller who was selling defective Dobermans. Winona's eyes were too light and her palate was cleft. Show dogs cost a thousand dollars. For Winona we paid a hundred. On the day we picked her up it was 106 degrees in the outdoor pen where she was lying on her side, her belly round as a softball, panting like she'd sprinted a mile. Katya held her on her lap for the drive back to Houston in my 1957 Chevrolet pickup. When I bought it from its original owner my dad asked why I'd get a car older than me. I opened the hood and pointed to the engine block. I said, Because I like things I can understand. The truck had five windows, two gas tanks, and after-market air-conditioning. Winona pressed her snout against the vent and smiled.

When she was seven months' pregnant, Katya took Winona to the vet for routine vaccines. The vet looked at Katya's belly and asked whether this was our first. She advised us to buy a doll to prepare Winona for the new arrival. You hear stories about Dobermans mauling babies. When Katya repeated the story to me that night I laughed. I said, People I don't get, but I am absolutely positive there is zero chance Winona will hurt our son. I didn't call him Lincoln, even though we had already decided on the name. There's no upside in tempting fate.

From the day we brought Lincoln home, Winona stood sentry at his crib. Way before Lincoln could crawl, he would reach his hand through the slats and poke his index finger into her eyes or grab ahold of her floppy ears and tug them like taffy. Winona shook her head and licked his hand and took a step back, and kept standing guard, just beyond his reach.

Peter liked to take Winona with him on his epic walks. He called us two nights before we were going to meet them in Galveston for the weekend. He said, *You're bringing Winona, right? I need to give that dog some hard pets.*

By this time I'd known Peter four years. We talked politics and history, physics and art. He loved music and theater and setting off at dawn with a daypack, a compass, a map, and not a plan. He taught me to windsurf and for my birthday bought Katya and me a week's worth of whitewater lessons at the Harvard of kayaking schools. He cherished the solitude. I preferred the adrenaline. We paddled together four or five times a year until I started running sections of rivers he was too prudent to descend.

The day before Thanksgiving the year before, we put our boats in the salt flats off the north side of Galveston Isle. We paddled into the marsh, too far from shore for anyone to walk. We turned a bend and there were a thousand birds, maybe more, standing in the shallows. They'd probably never seen a person here. They looked at us, curious but unafraid. I said, Wow.

Peter said, *Yes.*

We sat there and watched. He finally said, *I think boating might have made you an environmentalist.*

I said, Environmentalism is not a moral choice. It's just an aesthetic preference, like choosing chocolate over vanilla.

He did not turn to look at me. Staring at the birds he said, *You don't believe that.*

His first round of chemo was scheduled for the following week. When I asked him about it the eve before our trip to Galveston he was evasive. I said, Remember to bring your kayaking gear.

He said, *I'll try.*

The next morning before driving to the prison I took Winona for a run and a swim. When we came inside at six, Katya was already up, making tea. She said, I've been doing some reading. I think it's possible his tumor is a Merkel cell melanoma. If I am right, he needs to get radiation. If that's not what it is, I think immunotherapy is his best option. I'm going to call him at eight.

One thing I've learned is that there are times you have to let the people you love hold on to hope the math rules out. To do that, you have to pretend not to worry. Honesty is important, but it pales next to support.

I said to Katya, Good. I told her his diet was high in antioxidants and low in fats. I told her those things even though I knew there was no evidence it meant anything at all. I used the term *dysplastic nevi* not to impress her, but to sound like I had done enough research to make my endorsement of her opinion worth respecting.

I didn't tell her what Peter had said to me before he hung up the night before. He had said, *There aren't any surprises in life. Surprises are what we call things that happen when we aren't paying attention.*

■ ■ ■

drove to the prison to see Waterman for the first time. A few years ago, prison officials found more than fifty cell phones on death row, one for every seven inmates. They conducted the cell-to-cell search because one of the prisoners used his phone to call a state senator known for being tough on crime. Here's something I've learned: The death penalty cannot deter crime, and if you want to understand why, all you need to know is that death row inmates are the kind of people who use phones they are not supposed to have to dial up the home number of a state official and interrupt his dinner hour to complain about their treatment.

The phones, of course, were provided by guards who got up to a thousand dollars apiece for them. They weren't discovered for years because prisoners are clever. If these guys used the ingenuity they show in prison on the outside, half of them would be successful entrepreneurs. To thwart strip searches, one of the prisoners hid his phone up his rectum. An X ray finally revealed it. We spent half a day in my office discussing whether we were obligated to inform prison officials when our clients called us. (The vote was split.) Because of the scandal, the prison entrance was modified to resemble airport security. Now, your shoes and personal possessions are scanned, and everyone—civilians as well as guards—has to walk through a metal detector. Then a guard pats you down and looks at the bottoms of your shoeless feet.

That day, when I lifted my right foot for him to have a look, Officer Monroe laughed. My sock had a hole. He said, I thought you attorneys made the big bucks. Two weeks later when I was at the prison again he gave me a brown paper sack. Inside was a new pair of navy blue dress socks. They still had the price tag. He said, Receipt's in the bag, in case you want to take 'em back and get a new color or different size. When I thanked him he laughed.

After passing through two gates, two razor-wire-topped fences, and three electronic doors, I reached the visiting area. The visiting area has two long, shelflike surfaces, divided by metal partitions, where visitors sit and talk to the inmates on a phone. Officer Scott led me to an attorney booth. It's a space the size of an airplane lavatory where lawyers can visit privately with their clients. Before she closed the door behind me she said, Let me know if you need anything.

I sat there for forty minutes waiting for a team of three guards to bring Waterman in. Prison officials make a game of wasting lawyers' time, but they are neither bright nor creative, and once you know their tactics of passive aggression, they are easy to thwart. I keep a book in my car in case of traffic jams, and a stack of death penalty cases I need to read in the satchel I take with me to death row. I had made it through four of them when I heard a high-pitched lispy voice that reminded me of a young Mike Tyson. Waterman said something as they were unshackling him. The two white guards on his left and his right laughed. The black sergeant, who was two steps behind, didn't. He made eye contact with me and nodded.

Waterman was wearing a prison-issued white cotton jumpsuit

with the letters DR stenciled on the back in black. His hair was cut very short and he was cleanly shaved. He had a scar that slanted diagonally across the right nostril of his flattened nose and a teardrop tattooed below the outside corner of his left eye. He picked up the phone on his side of the glass and looked at the earpiece. He spat on it and used a corner of his jumpsuit to wipe it clean. Like many death row inmates, Waterman appeared to be a germaphobe. He held the phone to his ear and waited for me to speak. I told him who I was.

He said, Very nice to meet you, sir. His teeth were even and paper white.

I was there to introduce myself, tell him who would be working with me on this case, and give him some idea what we would be trying to do.

A death penalty case has four layers. First comes the trial and the state court appeal. Next comes a state court habeas proceeding. Then there is a federal habeas appeal. Finally there is everything else, all the last-minute freneticism when death penalty lawyers try to think of anything they can to save their client's life. Waterman's case was at the third stage. Before President Clinton signed the Antiterrorism and Effective Death Penalty Act, known to death penalty lawyers as AEDPA, you could take as long as you wanted to file the appeal at the third stage. Now you have less than a year. And in general, the only issues you can raise in the federal habeas appeal are issues that were raised in one of the two previous stages. If an inept lawyer neglects to raise a promising issue at an early stage, other lawyers will not be able to raise it later. I explained all this to Waterman. He nodded and said, Yes, I understand.

Waterman's trial lawyer had tried to persuade the jury that Miss McClain was already dead when Waterman shot her, and that he should therefore not be sentenced to death. What Waterman did was horrific, the lawyer had said, maybe even unforgivable, but if you kick a dead person, you can't be guilty of killing her. It was not necessarily a bad argument. The trial lawyer's mistake was that he had not hired an expert to determine whether Miss McClain was in fact already dead when Waterman shot her. We did. The pathologist reviewed photographs and lab reports and concluded the first shot had killed Miss McClain instantly. My plan was to focus on the trial lawyer's mistake and try to persuade a court that if he had just hired an expert, the jury would not have convicted Waterman of murder. We had already started interviewing jurors, and one had told us that she would have voted to convict Waterman of a lesser crime if she had known that.

Cara and Jeffrey are the two lawyers who work with me. They are in their mid-twenties, smart, tireless, and passionate. When I told them my plan, they were not enthusiastic. Jeffrey said, Even if he didn't kill her, he was still there. He was a party to the murder.

Most states, including Texas, have laws that allow everyone who participates in a crime to receive the maximum allowable punishment. It is known as the law of parties. If two guys rob a bank, and one sits in the car while the other goes inside, and the guy who goes inside kills a teller, the getaway driver can be sentenced to death. In fact, he can be sentenced to death even if the actual killer is not.

I said, That's true, but the jury did not convict him on that theory. They convicted him for causing Miss McClain's death. If the first shot killed her, then Waterman did not cause her death.

Cara said, Will anybody care about that? It's such a legalistic point.

I said, We're lawyers. All our points are legalistic.

She said, That's not what I mean. I mean it's not our best argument.

What's better?

Cara and Jeffrey wanted to focus on the fact Waterman was no longer dangerous. In other death penalty states, the jurors who decide whether to sentence someone to death consider many factors, including whether they think the defendant will be dangerous in the future if he is not executed. In Texas, that's the only factor the jury assesses. But juries are often wrong when they try to predict someone's future behavior. One study has them being wrong 95 percent of the time. Cara and Jeffrey wanted to structure our appeal around the fact the jury had been wrong in Waterman's case. From the day he got to prison he had been a model inmate. His only disciplinary infractions were for masturbating in his cell.

I said, The guy coldcocked a nurse at a gas station and two days later shot an elderly woman for her Cadillac and said *That's how you smoke a bitch*. He's pretty much the poster child of a callous cruel bastard. The judges aren't going to interview him. They'll just read the transcript. They might not even do that. They might just read the excerpts the attorney general puts in its brief. That's all they'll see, period. They're not capable of getting past that comment even if they're willing to, which they're not. On top of which, the issue was not raised in state habeas. We're barred from raising it.

Jeffrey started to lay out the argument for why we might be able to raise it anyway. It was not a bad argument, but I'd heard it before. In fact, I helped write it. I said, I know the logic. The answer is no. Sometimes you show weakness by saying too much. We've got one strong argument here. Every crappy claim we raise alongside it makes it more and more dilute.

My office was quiet. I picked up my Super Ball and bounced it on the desk. I looked at Jeffrey and Cara. They were willing me to change my mind. I zinged the ball off the wall. I said, I don't think we can win this case by humanizing Waterman.

Cara was pursing her lips like a fish. She said, But Eddie *is* a human being. I raised my eyebrows but said nothing. It takes a while for the young lawyers who work for me to realize the judges we have to persuade aren't the choir. In fact, they aren't even members of the church. She'd learn soon enough.

Meanwhile, Jeffrey was shifting his weight back and forth, right to left, left to right. There was nothing more to say, but they weren't leaving. I said, Tell you what. Write up the issue. We can hang on to it for Plan B.

I gave Waterman an abbreviated version of the conversation I'd had with Cara and Jeffrey. He said, We was all pretty fucked up. It ain't no excuse or nothin'. I ain't sayin' it is. I just want you to know.

Besides wanting to introduce myself and tell Waterman our plan, I was also there to learn something about him. After many years in prison, he still looked like a linebacker. Death row inmates do not have access to weights or a gym. He must have been doing a thousand push-ups a day. His rapport with the guards was good. He said, I'm realistic. Lotta guys been killed since I got here.

Like many inmates, he said *killed* instead of *executed*.

While I had been waiting for him I did the math in my head. I figured he'd be dead in twenty-eight months, but I planned to keep that calculation to myself. I said, We're going to do everything we can.

He broke off eye contact and looked behind me, over my right shoulder. Officer Scott was standing outside the closed door. Waterman could see her through the glass. He smiled at her. She tapped on the door and I opened it. Death row has vending machines filled with sodas, sandwiches, chips, and candy. Visitors can buy food for the inmates. They put change in the machine, and the guards remove the items and pass them to the prisoners. She wanted to know whether I was planning to buy something for Waterman. I wasn't. I was anxious to finish the visit and go home. I told Waterman I had to leave in a minute but I could get him some food he could take back to his cell. He said, Nah. But thanks anyway. I told Officer Scott next time. She waved at Waterman and closed the door. He looked at me again and said, It wasn't my idea to shoot the lady, but I didn't try to stop him or nothin'. It all happened pretty fast.

I nodded. He said, All right. Just so you know what happened.

He chewed on his lower lip. He was leaning forward, his forearms on the shelf, his chin nearly touching the back of his hand. He said, You know that lady who said I beat her at the gas station? I said I did. He said, That wadn't me. Ain't gonna say who did it but it wadn't me. I was driving the car. I looked at him, saying nothing. He said, Maybe it don't matter. But it wadn't me.

I said, I'll check it out.

He said, I know it don't mean nothin', but it wadn't me. I ain't got no reason to blow smoke. Only reason I'm sayin' something is so you know.

I asked about his family. He had written his daughter five times over the past two years, but she had not written back. He said, Her momma don't want her to have nothin' to do with me. I don't really blame her. When I got here, they shoulda executed me. That's still who she thinks I am.

He shook his head. One of the guards behind him said something. Waterman put the phone down, turned halfway around, said something back, and laughed. He looked at the phone's earpiece then held it up to his other ear.

I said, What's that about?

He said, Aw, they're saying I'm gonna be skinny next time they see me. Got a chess game goin' with the captain. Loser buys the winner ten candy bars.

I said, You play chess?

He said, Picked it up when we was back at Ellis.

He was referring to the Ellis Unit, where death row inmates were housed several years ago. When they were at Ellis, they had group exercise or recreation. Waterman's next-door neighbor had been a middle-age white guy who killed his family for insurance money. He'd grown up in New York playing speed chess in Morningside Park. He taught Waterman how to play on a checkerboard using animal crackers for chess pieces. Waterman read at a seventh-grade level, but in his cell he kept a shelf of chess books and studied the diagrams. He said, I won once and he won once. Two draws. This is the decider.

I said, If I need someone inside to say something good about you, will the captain talk to me?

Waterman said, Don't know. He might. What for?

I said, In case we have to go to Plan B.

I closed my notebook and packed up to go. He said, Can I ask you a question ain't got nothin' to do with my case? I told him sure. He said, I think the lady we killed has a nephew. Can I tell him I'm sorry?

■ ■ ■

P eople think death row inmates find religion because of their proximity to the gurney. That's not it at all. They feel remorse because they cannot escape what they have wrought. They spend twenty-three hours a day in a box the size of your closet with no television, no computer, and no iPods. They get Christian radio stations and visits from chaplains who read them all the commandments they've violated. They are not bibliophiles, if they can even read at all. They have all day every day to do nothing except think about the myriad ways they've screwed up their lives. There's not a single thing to distract them from what they have done, and what they've done is lose their own families and destroy another. Death row inmates do not become remorseful because they are scared to die. They aren't scared to die. Some of them prefer it, in fact. They become remorseful because they don't have enough space to evade the enormity of their deeds.

One thing I've learned is that the worst fate that can befall someone who has done something truly horrible is to be forced to face it alone, all day every day, without excuse, distraction, or surcease.

I told Waterman of course he could.

He said, Thank you for coming to see me, sir, and for trying to help.

■ ■ ■

I no longer dream of ruin. It used to wake me at 2 A.M. and keep me up until dawn. Now when I shudder in fear of failure, I am always wide awake. It might be early evening or midafternoon. I am kissing my wife or holding my son. I'm petting the dog. I am driving home from the prison, unable to leave the smell of broken lives behind.

Broken lives do have a smell. They reek of melting plastic and rotten eggs. It is an odor chlorine cannot mask. I can't outdrive it and I can't ignore it. It clings to me until I step into my kitchen and finally smell home.

Katya and I have a friend whose two children hate him. It's his opinion, not ours. He told us over dinner how he worked eighteen-hour days to provide for them, and they resented him for never being home. He swallowed without chewing and guzzled red wine like it was a competition. He seemed wistful, and resigned. My clients have the opposite problem. Their dizzyingly dysfunctional homes would have been better without the parents. But I have to think some of these moms and dads loved their kids as much as my wife and I love our son. Something just got in the way.

Lincoln will not become one of my clients, I know that, and I will not become our friend. I also know why: It is a mixture of will and fate. What I don't know, what I wish I knew, are the proportions.

Katya was at a budget meeting at Lincoln's school. Maria was making Lincoln's dinner. She's been with us since Lincoln was six weeks old. Eight years later, Lincoln did not need a nanny anymore, but she had become part of the family. I told her I'd take over the cooking and see her tomorrow. Lincoln said, Hasta mañana, Nana.

From Katya he learned to share his meals with Winona. When Lincoln was young, he couldn't pronounce her name either. He said, Dada, watch how Nonie won't eat my grill cheese, even if I put it on the floor right in front of her, until I tell her it's okay.

I said, Linco, a grilled cheese is not good for her.

He said, But she likes it.

I said, Sometimes people like things that aren't good for them.

He said, You mean like you smoking cigars?

I said, Go ahead and feed her, amigo.

And I thought, The difference is that I do the cost-benefit analysis for myself, whereas you are doing it for Winona.

But what is the difference, really? The calculation is either right or wrong, and it doesn't have anything to do with who does the math. We have this notion that certain people are entitled to make decisions, but maybe it's completely backward. Maybe Waterman should get to decide on his own litigation strategy and Katya should get to decide her dad's treatment regimen. If everyone's identity is a function of all the perspectives of the people who know her, then the more people you know, the less your life is yours. When Waterman dies, there will be a news story. When Peter dies, people will cry.

Until I met Katya, I wanted to live in the middle of nowhere with just a piano, a bike, a dog, good whiskey, and my books. Even after we married, I could still see the piece of land I almost bought, could still see myself sitting beside the two-acre spring-fed pond. When our son came along, the picture lost its focus.

Lincoln said, Okay. Then will you help me brush her teeth?

I watched him tear off pieces of sandwich the size of grapes. Winona would gently take the sandwich pieces with her front teeth and savor each bite. When there was none left she licked the corner of his mouth. I said, I think she found one last crumb on your face.

He said, No, Dada. She was saying thank you.

After he finished dinner we went to the grocery store. At the checkout line he asked if I would buy him two candy bars. I told him no, he had just had dessert. He begged and cajoled. From the time he was in preschool his teachers knew him as a negotiator. He said, How about one? I relented.

A woman wearing black leggings and a sweatshirt was standing behind me. She said, Are you ever going to tell him no?

I turned around. Her cart was piled high and overflowing with gallons of milk and dozens of eggs, like my mom's used to be. I said, Probably not, ma'am, but give me your phone number and I'll call you if I change my mind. I stared at her until she pulled a *People* magazine off the shelf and pretended to read.

Lincoln liked to push the buttons on the credit card scanner. After I swiped my card I said, Okay, Lincoln, time to press the enter button.

The checkout clerk looked at me oddly. She said, You named your kid after a car?

Most death penalty lawyers I know don't have children. Maybe they're like I used to be, wanting to own their lives, not understanding it's better not to. So the work fills their void. Their clients are their kids. It makes them completely committed to saving lives, but

27

leaves them clueless about what it means to be a mom or dad, about how easy it is to fuck up another human being. After our earlier strategy meeting, when Cara who had not yet met Waterman called him by his Christian name, I told her it is important to keep some distance between herself and our clients. She said, Why?

While Lincoln put on his pajamas, Katya read him a story. I said, Do you want me to help you floss your teeth or can you do it yourself?

He said, I would like some help, please.

I said, Really?

He said, Yes, Dada. It's a great opportunity for you.

Winona climbed into his bed. Katya and I walked downstairs, hand in hand. She said, Any bad news today?

I said, Well, I met with Waterman. I think Cara and Jeffrey might have been right.

■　■　■

Angry people are bitter, and bitter people are cold. Peter was angry because the cosmos cheated. He had a forty-year plan: two decades of toil—one he loved, one he hated—followed by two decades of play. He had a new sailboat, a new windsurfer, two new kayaks, hiking shoes for every terrain, sleeping bags for every climate, waterproof maps for every locale. He had a spiral notebook listing the places he planned to see. His budget's precision would have left a corporate CFO agog. Anyone else would've thought Peter was Robert Crumb.

After the surgery to remove the mass, when the pathology report came back, the doctor said, I think what we have here is a subcutaneous metastasis. But it is a very unusual mass. I am not entirely certain it is malignant.

In English: Maybe it was not cancer at all. If it was, the tumor the surgeon had removed might not have been Peter's first. The cancer might have started elsewhere. If the lump was a metastasis with an unknown primary tumor, there was an 85 to 95 percent chance Peter would be dead in five years. But if the tumor had simulated a cutaneous metastatic melanoma and was in fact the first appearance of cancer, there was an 85 percent chance he'd be alive in eight years if he pursued other therapies. His doctor needed to know which was which. He told Peter, We need to take some additional lymph nodes so we know how to proceed.

We were all sitting on the deck, waiting for the coals to burn down so I could put the redfish on the grill. Nights were coming early, and the sky was already pink. I got up to light a cigar and went to stand downwind. Katya asked, What does that mean, Papa?

He said, *I am not sure. I did not ask. He was very busy.*

She looked across the deck at me, pointed an imaginary gun at her head, and pulled the trigger. She said, What time is the operation next week?

He said, *Katya, dear, I think I am not going to have it.*

What?

If it is cancer and has already spread, there is nothing to do. If it is cancer and has not already spread, there is nothing to do. If it is not cancer at all, there is nothing to do.

Katya opened her mouth to speak but said nothing. She turned and walked inside. I told Peter I'd be right back and followed her in. She was in the kitchen gripping the counter. Her arms were shaking. She said, He's my papa. He's talking to me like a scientist.

Katya was still in the first stage of grief: denial. She said, It might not even be cancer. If it's not, he needs to know that. If it is and has already spread, he needs to know how to fight it.

I said, Before every execution, when I'm in my office at five o'clock waiting for the Supreme Court to call, I'm sure we are going to win.

She said, There's a difference between optimism as a defense mechanism and optimism as a strategy. Your attitude doesn't have any influence on the world. Mine might matter. His will definitely matter.

A friend and colleague of mine had recently learned she had stage IV breast cancer. The night before we drove to Galveston we had dinner with an oncologist and told her the story about my friend. She said, The five-year survival rate for women with stage IV breast cancer is 17 percent. Don't tell anyone I said this, but as best I can tell, the major difference between them and the other 83 percent is will.

I looked at Katya. It was like giving crack to an addict. Later that night I said, K, she might have confused cause and effect.

Katya said, And she might not have.

We ate on the deck so the crashing waves could mask our silence. Katya and Irmi hurried off to sleep. Peter and I stayed outside sipping Haitian rum as rich as cognac. There was no moon. He had to talk loudly over the surf. He said, *What I did not say to Katya is that there is no reason to take out lymph nodes because I have already decided not to have more chemotherapy. I can feel there is cancer everywhere. I finally understand the metaphor of cancer as an invading army. I can either spend the rest of my life trying to extend my life, or I can spend the rest of my life living my life. What would you do?*

I said, My entire life consists of trying to put off the end.

He said, *That's for others. What if it were you?*

If I told him to do nothing, I'd be betraying my wife. If I told him to fight, I'd be urging futility. My deeply held philosophy, given a choice between the lesser of evils, is to choose neither.

I said, Your family would like it if you would stick around as long as possible.

I congratulated myself for threading the needle. Some people would just call it cowardice.

■ ■ ■

31

C ontrary to what you might believe, resignation and will are not opposite sides of the same coin. They're adversaries in the struggle every human being facing crisis or despair confronts. You'll hear about the petite woman who sees the car fall off the jack and land on her son, and she rushes outside and lifts it off him like a cartoon. But when two officers wearing dress blues arrive to tell her that her boy, now a lance corporal in the United States Marine Corps, was blown to smithereens when his APC rolled over an IED outside Fallujah, and she waits until they leave before washing down a bottle of pilfered Valium with a fifth of JD, her obituary will be a single column inch on an inside page of the local news. Her DNA is exactly the same now as it was then. It's just a different team that's winning.

When Lincoln was in second grade, the big event of the school year was Famous Persons Day. The students spent six weeks researching a famous person of their choosing and writing a report they would have seven minutes to read. Lincoln decided not to write about Abraham Lincoln. Too obvious, he said.

Largely because he likes chocolate, he chose to report on Milton Hershey. Hershey started the Hershey Chocolate Company in 1894.

Every day a new book about Hershey came in the mail. Lincoln downloaded titles onto his reader and stuffed his backpack with books from the school library. He made notes as he read and organized them before bed.

Two nights before the program, we were sitting in the library. Lincoln was working on Hershey and petting the dog, Katya and I were reading. Suddenly Lincoln got up and ran to the bathroom. We heard him retching. Winona trotted over to check. He came back into the library wiping his mouth and said, I think I am getting a little sick. I'm going to go upstairs and take my temperature.

When he came back down he said, It's just a little high, just a hundred.

He went into the kitchen and came back with a cup of ice water and a bowl. He said, Just in case I throw up again.

Three times over the next two hours he interrupted his reading to throw up into the bowl. He'd carry it to the kitchen, rinse it out, and come back. He'd drink a swallow of water and go on like a normal day. Winona was pacing a circle. I was looking for the phone number of my pediatrician cousin. When he went to bed he said, I hope I feel better tomorrow.

The next morning he came downstairs and said, I'm still not feeling my best so is it okay if I skip breakfast? I don't want to throw up in my classroom. Winona and I drove him to school. I told him I hoped he felt better soon. He heaved his backpack onto his shoulders and said, Me too. He petted Winona on the head and headed off to class, bouncing on the balls of his feet like a sprinter, an advertisement for happiness.

At my office Cara was waiting for me with two students. I said, Y'all are here early.

Cara said, We got all the school records. Eddie was absent more than he was there. How did he ever graduate from one grade to the next? Shouldn't somebody from the school have called his house and figured out he was living by himself? Why didn't the trial lawyer use any of this stuff?

I said, The trial lawyer didn't use it because he probably didn't know, and he probably didn't know because he didn't care. Which also, by the way, explains the school administrators. That's what you showed up so early to tell me?

Cara said, No. We got affidavits from four more jurors who said they would have voted to convict of a lesser offense if they had known the victim was probably already dead when Eddie shot her.

I said, Five out of twelve. That's fantastic. I told you this claim was a winner. One day you'll probably start listening to me.

■　■　■

Driving home I called Peter. He had decided not to have more chemo. He said, *It makes me too ill to contemplate. But I will have the operation to remove three more lymph nodes. That way, at least we will know how long we have.* I asked him how Katya had responded. He said, *She is very smart. I know she is able to understand boundaries, to apprehend the boundary between my life and hers; she simply does not care about it.*

I said, I think you are confusing your physical existence with your life. They're not the same, and their boundaries aren't either.

He said, *Hmmm.*

I told Katya about our conversation. She said, He told me *we* made a decision, as if he has actually consulted us. I bet he hasn't even said anything to Mama. He's too angry to be rational, and too scared to admit it.

I said, Maybe he is being rational.

She said, If you don't have the facts, it isn't rational. Even if you get the right answer, it's just luck. I said nothing. She said, But if the luck is good, I won't complain. She asked about Waterman and I told her about the jurors. She said, Maybe we'll all have good luck this time, a different kind of story for once.

The next morning Winona and I got up early and went out for a run. When we got home an hour later, the eastern sky was bleeding from black to blue. We waited outside for Hector, who was three houses away. He saw us on the driveway and handed me the newspapers instead of tossing them on the porch. He said, Buenos días, señor.

Hector and I had known each other for a while. On a Thursday morning four years before, a cat streaked across the street two feet in front of his truck's driver side tire and never had a chance. Winona and I were jogging toward him as it happened, and saw it backlit like an old home movie. Hector jumped out saying Dios mío, Dios mío. He saw me and said, No es mi culpa. I told him I knew it wasn't his fault. He bent down. The cat was breathing, a trickle of blood spilling from its open mouth. He asked if I knew whose cat it was. I didn't. He picked up the inert animal and put it on the passenger seat. He looked at me and said, No se preoccupe. Tengo que ir al medico. Yo regreso.

A man who interrupts his paper route and risks termination from a job he cannot afford to lose to save the life of a cat he could easily ignore is a man I want to know. I wrote my cell number down on a notepad he kept on his dashboard and asked him to call me and tell me what happened.

When I saw him that morning four years later I said, Gracias, Hector. ¿Hay unas noticias buenas hoy? It was an inside joke. He had once seen me on TV talking about a case of someone he knew. My client was a Mexican kid named Walter who'd stolen a car with two other kids. I call them kids because they were seventeen. One of the other kids shot and killed the car's owner, an Air Force colonel who'd served in Iraq. All three were sentenced to death. In a case called *Roper v. Simmons*, the Supreme Court ruled that states cannot execute people who are under eighteen when they commit murder, but *Simmons* was decided in 2005. Hector's neighbor was executed in 2004. I had asked both the Supreme Court and the governor to intervene. The interviewer asked me whether I was optimistic. I told him of course not. The news for my clients is almost always bad. The next morning Hector asked me why I keep doing it then. I said, Por que siempre yo espero que la próxima vez sea diferente. He nodded. I do always expect today to be different. Every death penalty lawyer in Texas does.

He laughed and said, Yo no se. The cat whose life he'd saved stretched across his lap in the front seat. He told me his daughter was going to transfer from community college to the university where I teach. I told him to make sure she stops by my office to say hello. He said, Claro. Gracias, señor.

He started to drive off and I said, Un momentito. Una cosa mas. I handed him an envelope with a twenty-dollar bill inside. I said, Feliz Navidad y el año nuevo.

Without opening it he said, Thank you, mister.

Inside Katya was already sitting in the kitchen sipping tea. I asked why she was already up. She said, Were you talking to somebody out there?

I said, I gave Hector the twenty dollars for Christmas. I've had it in my pocket every morning for a week. His daughter's transferring to UH.

She said, Wow. That's great.

She drank a swallow of tea. Winona had lain down beside her, cooling herself on the slate floor. Katya put her right foot on Winona's chest and said, I've been doing research. I know he won't ask the doctor any questions so I'm just going to learn it myself.

I sat down next to her. I draped my arm across her shoulders and pushed a strand of hair behind her ear. She was staring into her tea. She said, He's always been terrified of getting old. I think he sees this as his escape.

She had both hands wrapped around her mug. The sky was light now but we could still see a sliver of moon dropping in the western sky. We watched the sparrows and cardinals eat from our feeders and a squirrel pull a pomegranate from the tree. Katya said, They don't even like pomegranates. They rob us of pleasure and there isn't any offsetting benefit to anyone.

I said, Is that supposed to be a metaphor?

She said, No.

I topped off Winona's food bowl and put my coffeemaker on the stove.

Katya said, But it could be. She paused then added, I'm going to need you to help me get through to him.

I said, You figure out the treatment and I'll tie him to a chair and administer it myself.

She said, I'm not joking, Diablo.

I said, Neither am I.

■ ■ ■

That afternoon I drove up to Nacogdoches, a small East Texas town midway between Dallas and Houston, but closer to Shreveport in both distance and culture. Waterman's sister Hattie lived there with her husband and three kids on five acres in a weathered A-frame with a shaded deck. She worked a third shift cleaning classrooms and faculty offices at Stephen F. Austin University. Her husband operated an X ray and ultrasound machine at the local hospital. I hadn't called to let her know I was coming.

I drove all the way up to the porch, scattering a dozen or so goats and chickens that were pecking at the bare ground. I left the dog in the car. I heard water running and knocked on the frame of the flimsy door. Hattie shouted who is it from inside and I said it was her brother's lawyer. She opened the door wearing latex kitchen gloves and a house robe. She peeled off the gloves and said, 'Scuse me. I been doin' the dishes. I told her my name and apologized for arriving unannounced. I asked her if we could talk. She said, You mind if we sit outside?

She lit a cigarette with a plastic lighter and shook one out of the pack at me. I told her no thank you. She turned her head to exhale a stream of smoke away from me then said, So what you need with me? I told her I was just trying to learn everything I could about her brother, and he had told me she knew him better than anyone. Hattie said, I reckon that's prob'ly true.

She told me she'd grown up in Longview. Her mother was a drunk who died while she was six months' pregnant with her second kid when she ran her car into a flooded creek near Kilgore and drowned. Hattie was seven. She said, Ain't you gonna write any of these things down?

I told her someone in my office would put all the names on a family tree for me, that I was just there to get an impression of what Waterman's early life had been like. She nodded and continued. She told me her father drove an eighteen-wheeler when he wasn't in prison. After Hattie's mother died, he asked a neighbor, Johanna, to look after Hattie when he was gone. Johanna was sixteen. She had a son named Jojo who was two. At the time, Hattie didn't know that Jojo was her half brother.

A week before Hattie turned nine, Waterman was born. Her father failed a third drug test and got fired. She doesn't know what happened, but one day, Johanna, Jojo, and Waterman were gone.

I said, What do you mean, gone?

She said, I come home from school and ain't no one home. Still weren't nobody home when I went to sleep or when I woke up the next morning. Just gone. When he got back with the truck I asked him where they was and he tole me don't worry about it.

Hattie later learned her father had beaten Johanna so viciously he broke her jaw in three places and cracked four of her teeth. Johanna apparently refused to press charges, but she did take her two boys, and she left her abuser behind. As far as Hattie knew,

Waterman's mother and father had never spoken to each other again.

Johanna worked at a fried chicken place. She asked Hattie if she could look after Jojo and Waterman when she went to work, and Hattie said sure.

Sometime later—she told me it was a few days, but I did not entirely trust her memory on the timing—Hattie got home from school and found a woman named Cheryl watching TV. Cheryl was Hattie's dad's new wife. She moved into the tiny house with four kids, three girls and a boy. One afternoon when Hattie got home from school, Cheryl accused her of having sex with her father and pulled out a gun.

Hattie started going to Johanna's house to look after Jojo and Waterman over there. Some nights she'd sleep on the floor in a room where the two boys shared a single bed.

Johanna was a crack addict. She brought home leftover biscuits, fries, and chicken thighs for her boys. Hattie wasn't sure the kitchen held a refrigerator.

Hattie told me Johanna would talk to herself and walk down the middle of the street slashing the air in front of her face with a knife like she was slicing through a wall. I asked her whether she said anything to her father. She'd smoked the cigarette down to the filter. She tossed the butt into an old flowerpot and lit another. She was thirty-seven years old. She shook her head, weary, like she was tired of explaining something complicated to a simpleton in a language he didn't understand. She said, No sir. There wouldn't a been no point to that.

Jojo killed himself. He was ten years old. Shot himself through the heart with a gun Hattie didn't know he had. If it was possible, Johanna got worse. She'd stay in her bedroom with the curtains drawn twenty hours a day, watching television, smoking PCP-laced cigarettes, and drinking cheap vodka from a plastic bottle. She either got fired or quit the job at the chicken place. Police drove out to the house at least twice when neighbors heard her screams through the plywood walls. I said, What happened on the day the police took her away?

Calling Waterman by his first name she said, Eddie called me and said Mommy was trying to hurt him. I asked him where he was at and he said in a bathroom. I told him to stay where he was and I'd be right over, and I called 911 and got on my bike. He must have called the police before me 'cause they was already there when I rode up. Some lady police was sittin' there talkin' to Eddie. I told her I was his sister and after a few minutes they tole me I could take him on home. We come back to the house but Cheryl said there wadn't no room for us. So we just stayed at Johanna's. They eventually locked us out but it didn't matter 'cause by then Eddie wasn't living there no more.

I knew this story already, but hearing it told by someone who saw it made me dizzy. It wrung the hope right out of me. It made me think the world is completely beyond our capacity to change, that we've created problems too big to fix. I thought about saying nice meeting you, getting up, and walking away. She said, You okay, mister?

I said, Did you go to Eddie's trial?

She said, Some days I did. When I could get off work. I had my own kids by then.

I said, Did you testify?

I knew the answer, but I asked anyway. She said, No. I asked her why not. She said, I told his lawyer I wanted to try to help but he said there wasn't nothin' I could do.

I said, Nice meeting you, Hattie. Thanks for your time. May I call you again if I need to?

She said, Course you can. Eddie's my brother.

■   ■   ■

Each of the three second-grade classes had fifteen students. Almost all their parents were there, and lots of grandparents too. The head of the lower school introduced the teachers, who were sitting in the front row. There were at least 150 people in the room.

Lincoln had written his report about Hershey on 5-by-7 lined index cards, but he'd practiced so much he knew the speech by heart. He would flip the cards without looking down, knowing where each ended and the next began. When it was his turn, he walked to the microphone, looked down at his notes, and said, Milton Snavely Hershey was born on September 13, 1857, in Cherry Church, Pennsylvania. Katya and I were beaming.

Just over two minutes in, he glanced down at his notes and paused. He was suddenly silent. He seemed confused. As it happened, several of the index cards had stuck together. When he intended to flip one, he had actually flipped three. The packed house was watching him saying nothing.

He realized what had happened. He pulled the cards apart, flipped back to his place, and resumed, his voice strong, his demeanor unaffected. If I told you those few seconds felt like ten minutes, and if you are a parent, you will undoubtedly know what I mean. The episode actually lasted fourteen seconds. I know this because I timed it when I watched the video for the seventh time. It was a display of poise I still remember all these years later, like it happened just now. On his report card that semester, his teacher, Mrs. Goldberg, wrote, *His poise and confidence in delivery—and recovery—gave me chills.*

There are moments, I think, when parents look at their children and wish they could do some things better. It's why I keep pushing Lincoln to go to wrestling camp. And then there are moments when parents look at their children and know they have just witnessed something they could never do. I watch that video again and again, and every time I experience awe.

I remembered Famous Persons Day on my drive back to town. How does a child become a kid who calmly makes two phone calls while his deranged mother is kicking down the door? How does that same kid become a young man who commits murder?

Or maybe the question should be: How does that kid not?

I stopped for gasoline in Shepherd, just south of Livingston, where Waterman was in his cell on death row, and when the cashier asked me if I needed anything else, I said, Yeah. I bought two bottles of Pacifico and sat down on the curb. It was nearly dusk.

Across the street a black man wearing a toque was tending to a smoker perched on a gooseneck trailer parked next to a wooden shack the size of an outhouse. He was wearing denim overalls and a butcher's smock and was holding a pair of tongs as long as a baseball bat. I walked over and asked him what was good. He said, Everything's good. He pronounced it *evra-tang*. I bought two quails and six brisket tacos, shredded meat wrapped in flour tortillas, covered with diced onions and pickled jalapeños. I asked for the fresh salsa on the

45

side. He asked, Spicy or spicier? I told him I'd take the hottest stuff he had. He put a pint-size Styrofoam cup in with my food. He said, It's gonna make you cry.

I called Katya and told her I was bringing dinner home. She said, What's the matter?

I said, Nothing.

She said, Uh-huh.

One thing I've learned is that just because you can successfully lie to yourself doesn't mean you're not completely transparent to the people you love. Of course, it's one thing to learn something. It's another to change. I said, I'll tell you about it when I get home.

But that night I didn't. After Katya and I hung up, Peter called our house to report the lymph nodes were full of cancer, and spots had appeared on his liver. Katya said to me, When I begged him to have surgery, he told me he would give it the *most serious consideration.* It was like talking to a stranger. Then he thanked me and hung up the phone.

■ ■ ■

*A*lthough I know the difference between a positive and a negative, I do not know how to weigh them. How much value should I give to Irmi and Katya's certainty the operation should proceed? If I permit the surgery, I am also tacitly agreeing to additional chemo, for without the poison, the operation makes no sense.

I called the surgeon, who did not call me back. I told his nurse I wanted him to confirm my calculations. If I undergo a complete hepatic resection that removes all the metastatic disease, there is a one-in-three chance I will be alive in three years, a one-in-five chance I will be alive in five. That assumes the liver metastases are isolated. Perhaps they are not, but maybe they are, and my fortune has finally changed. The oncologist also told me they can use the liver tumors to design a vaccine. There is no certainty it would work or that I will live long enough to try it. But even scientists can sometimes cling to faith.

If I do not have the surgery, I will be dead in four months.

I tell myself the math makes the decision for me, but I fear I am not at the center of this decision at all. I think I might be the opposite of Jim Bowie, and that is as bad as being him.

Enough. The decision is made. If all goes well, I will be in the hospital one week. Irmi and I check in tomorrow morning. The surgeon cuts me open tomorrow afternoon.

I am not telling you good-bye because I do not believe it is time.

■ ■ ■

im Bowie? That night at two his obscure reference finally sank in.

A week after the original pathology report, Peter and I spent the morning surfing a standing wave on a section of the Brazos River kayakers call Hidalgo Falls. The temperature was in the low 50s and a steady wind blew at ten from the north. Peter said, *This is glorious.* We had the river to ourselves.

When our shoulders were spent we drove into Navasota and bought brie and onion sandwiches and a six-pack of St. Arnold from a Muslim woman wearing a head scarf at a country store. We took the food to Stephen F. Austin State Park and parked under a canopy of hardwoods. We ate in the truck while a pileated woodpecker created a racket above. Peter said, *I will miss watching them.* He opened the door and leaned out, twisting his head to look up in the branches.

The bird flew off. I wanted to say something but feared I'd sound harsh. A sign listed events for Texas history month. Peter read it. He said, *They teach seventh graders that Jim Bowie was a hero at the Alamo. That's one view. The other is that he was a delusional romantic who sacrificed two hundred young men to his narcissistic fantasy. There's neither dishonor nor shame in recognizing the jig is up so others can live out the rest of their lives in joy.*

I looked at him and raised my eyebrows, hoping a gesture could say, What are you talking about? But if he could read my meaning, he ignored me.

I'd like you to do me another favor. I'd like it if you'd please tell Katya not to hold on too tight.

I said, Too tight? What's the matter with you? There's no such thing as too tight.

What do you tell your clients when they beg you to file something else an hour before their deaths?

That's not remotely the same thing.

Yes it is. It's exactly the same.

Winona needed to go outside. I sat at my computer and read. The median survival time for people with melanoma that has spread to one organ is seven months. As I saw it, that was Peter's most optimistic prognosis. If tumors had also spread to his lungs or brain, he was down to four months. If they had spread to both, he was down to two.

If the tumors were just in his liver, he had a one-in-three chance of still being alive in a year. In two organs, the odds were one in ten. In three, one in a hundred. I tried to reconstruct his math and couldn't. Was hope causing him to fudge the numbers? I closed the web browser and erased the history so Katya wouldn't see.

Winona banged open the door and came inside. She followed me to the stairs but wouldn't climb up. I said, Did you hurt yourself running? Later I would realize that was the first sign I missed. I scooped her in my arms and carried her up to bed. I lay there chasing sleep till nearly dawn. At six I whispered to Katya I'd see her later at the hospital, made a pot of coffee, and drove to the prison.

I was hoping to learn more about Waterman's childhood. The problem was, I couldn't find anyone besides Hattie who knew him when he was a child. Hattie told me first names of some neighborhood kids, but she didn't know where any of them were now. I thought Waterman might know. He said, Naw. I pretty much quit runnin' with anyone 'cept Demetrius and Harold 'round the time Mama left. I seen Hattie some. That's pretty much it.

I asked him whether he remembered how old he was when his mom was taken off to the asylum for the last time. He was looking at me but his eyes were flat. His hands were resting on the shelf, his fingers interlaced, like a penitent.

When I was in law school my best friend Jon and I had a running three-year argument about whether introspection is an indulgence of the bourgeoisie. Primo Levi says somewhere that the reason Jews in the concentration camps didn't commit suicide is they were too busy with the details of living. People who kill themselves have food in the pantry. I told Jon, We sit around in the dining hall discussing the meaning of life because we're going to be working fourteen-hour days and making seven figures by the time we're thirty. Rumination's a luxury. It might even be obscene.

Jon said, That's bullshit.

I made a note to call him that night and tell him he was right. It only took me fifteen years to notice.

Sitting there across from me, Waterman looked like a muscle-bound Romeo. I'm an expert at parrying anger, but sadness defeats me and makes me want to flee.

He said, I was six.

I saw the red veins in the whites of his eyes. I noticed his nostrils weren't the same size. Why was he wearing an earring? Is that allowed in the prison? I wanted to look away from him. But I couldn't.

He said, I got home and she was all hot, she ain't said why, and

I tole her hello and next thing she done was grab that butcher knife from outa the drawer and come after me. I hadn't done nothin'. I said, What'd I do, Momma? And she was just lookin' at me like she hadn't never seen me before. I ran around the table and she'd a caught me 'cept she tripped and fell. I locked myself in her bathroom and called 911 and then Hattie and they come and took her and she didn't never come home after that.

Here's something I've learned: When someone tells you something inconceivable, and you know for a fact he isn't insane, you need to give serious consideration to the possibility that the occurrence's very inconceivability is the bitter proof of how little you know.

Three times I had gone to the asylum where Waterman's mother lived. Calling it that is not hyperbole. I learned *One Flew Over the Cuckoo's Nest* was not a figment of Ken Kesey's imagination. On my final visit she told me she had not planned to kill all of him, only the part that had come from his daddy, the bad part. I asked her how she was going to do that. She said, It can be done, sir. I seen it done.

I said to Waterman, You know, one thing I've wondered is how much of that you really remember. I don't think I remember anything from when I was six years old. Maybe you just remember people telling you what happened.

Waterman shook his head slowly. He leaned toward me. He said, Professor—

I had told him half a dozen times to call me by my name. I said, You're still calling me Professor? But he didn't smile.

He said, Professor, I don't mean no disrespect, but when your momma chases you through the house with a knife that looks bigger than you are, screamin' at the top of her lungs she's gonna kill you, and you have to lock yourself in the bathroom and lean against the door and holler till the police get there…He paused and shook his head one time. I waited. He said, Sir, that's something you don't forget.

I pretended I needed to make a note so I had an excuse to look away. I know it is possible to destroy a child's capacity to empathize, but I am not sure the reverse is true. I said, Did you tell your trial lawyer this story?

No, sir.

Why not?

He didn't ask.

I said, Yeah, but you could have told him anyway.

He said, Don't really see why it woulda mattered. Didn't have nothing to do with what I done.

I asked him whether he was in touch with his mother. He said, Naw, not really. I hear she's doin' all right though. If you talk to her, tell her Eddie sends his love, okay?

■　■　■

Katya was at the hospital with her mom and her brother, Phil, who had flown in for the day. When I got there her dad had been in surgery for almost two hours. Doctors were removing 70 percent of his liver. They expected it to regrow within a few weeks. But up until they anesthetized Peter, the doctors were not on the same page. The oncologist had wanted to try another round of chemo to shrink the tumors before trying to remove them. The surgeon had said the tumors were clustered, so resection was appropriate, and Peter could get more chemo later. Katya asked about yttrium-90 microspheres. These are tiny beads containing low-level radiation that are injected into the arteries in the liver that feed individual tumors. The oncologist said, For tumors as large as your father's, we'd need a great deal of radiation, and the safe amount hasn't been clinically defined.

Katya said, What about ablation?

The oncologist looked like a politician trapped at a town hall meeting with a voter who understands the issues. He said, The tumors are too big.

It's surgery now and chemo later, or chemo now and surgery later. Which will it be?

A dozen clichés come to mind. A man with one watch knows what time it is; a man with two watches is never sure. And so on. In the middle of the Civil War, Lincoln's advisors were urging him to replace McClellan. Lincoln said a single bad general is better than two good ones. That might be wrong, but not for Peter. He was paralyzed by conflicting advice. The sniping among the doctors made Katya mad, but it just made Peter passive, and Irmi cry.

I hugged Katya and asked what the doctors said when her dad asked for their recommendation. She said, Has there ever been a patient less willing than Papa to ask his doctors for more information? I have a thousand questions and he won't ask even one. He thinks it's indecorous. That's his word. I think it's idiotic.

She wanted to cry, I could tell, but she didn't. She said, I talked to Mama and Phil and then I told them to operate.

When Katya, Lincoln, and I went to Germany to visit her family, we took a train south from Munich. She said, Watch how obsequious the passengers act toward the ticket collector. They defer to him because he's wearing a uniform. Can you imagine New Yorkers acting this way on the train to New Haven? If you want to understand the Holocaust, take a train in Bavaria.

We waited four more hours. I drank a gallon of coffee and ate two orders of fries from McDonald's, conveniently located on the hospital's first floor. It's like a vertical monopoly. You get sick on the first floor, and go upstairs for treatment.

When the surgeon came out, he told us Peter was in recovery, doing well, and that he believed he got all the tumors with good margins. Katya asked him when the next round of chemo would be scheduled. He told her to ask the oncologist. She said, When will he be coming around? The surgeon said he didn't know. I put my arm around her shoulders and could feel her instinct to shrug it off.

As soon as the surgeon walked out, she said, They sure are helpful here.

Half an hour later Katya and her mom went in to see her dad. There was a limit of two visitors per patient, so I went back to McDonald's for ice cream. I had managed about a pint's worth when Katya came down. She said, It's like he was waiting to pick a fight. Mama and I were talking about Thanksgiving and he said, *Ah yes, my last Thanksgiving.* I wanted to tell him he didn't have to come.

Did you?

No.

What did you say?

Nothing. I felt myself starting to cry.

Did he say anything?

No. He turned his head.

I said, Angry people say things they don't mean. He's angry. Give him time.

Being angry isn't license to be cold to the people who love you.

That's true, I said.

■   ■   ■

*B*etween the end and the beginning is the chaos. That was Metternich, the great German statesman. You know what he said next, when he heard about the revolution in France? He said his life was destroyed.

I have learned that one knows the precise moment when the chaos settles into order that leads like a rail to the preordained. For me it was just now. The doctor finally returned my call. They lost my liver.

They lost my goddamned liver.

So much for Katya's vaccine. Every time I resolve to do something proactive, the universe swats me down. I must have done something truly horrible to warrant this divine sanction, and I do not even know what it is.

■ ■ ■

One thing I've learned is there are times I know just from looking. What I don't know is whether it's because of the way they look, or the way I see. It doesn't matter. When I spotted Waterman's father from across the street, I knew exactly how our conversation would go.

I found him sitting in an aluminum lawn chair on the stoop of a sagging shotgun house in the heart of the Fifth Ward. I hadn't told him I was coming. I was wearing a suit. I was not interested in establishing rapport with him. I needed him to give me something. After a badge and a gun, a suit and tie are the next best thing. Before I could introduce myself he said, Who are you?

I told him my name and asked him his, and when he told me I said, Sir, I am a lawyer. I represent your son.

He said, Which boy's that?

I said, My client is your son Eddie Waterman. He rubbed his chin. He was smoking a cheroot that smelled like a ripe plantain. His teeth were the color of a root beer float. He turned his head to the left and spat off the porch.

He said, Been quite a while. What sorta trouble's he in?

I said, Your son is on death row.

He said, Who'd he done killed?

I explained that eight years ago Waterman and three others had killed a woman north of Dallas. I said one of the other men was also sentenced to death, one got ninety-nine years, the fourth got fifty years. He said, Boy's been over on death row for eight years? I said he had. He said, I ain't heard nothin' about it.

I said, Hattie didn't tell you?

He said, Ain't seen that one fer a spell.

I said, I'm hoping to talk to all Eddie's siblings, half or whole. Waterman's father furrowed his brow. I said, His brothers or sisters. I need to interview them.

Why you wanna be botherin' them?

I'm just trying to learn everything I can, sir. I'd like to get medical records for everyone in the family, and school records, too. I pulled a piece of paper from my satchel and said, This is a release. It authorizes me to obtain your medical records. Would you mind signing it?

He said, Me? What you need to know about me? I told him I was not looking for anything in particular. I was just collecting information. He said, Nobody did nothin' for me when I was inside. How'd Eddie get money to hire you?

He didn't give me any money. A judge appointed me to represent him.

Waterman's father took a deep drag from the cheroot. He opened a pocketknife and cleaned his thumbnail. He exhaled smoke through his nose. He said, I ain't been to no doctor recently.

I asked, Are you in touch with any of your children?

He said, Naw, not really. Not too much.

I held out the release again. He looked at it but made no move to take it. He said, I'm agonna have to think on it. You know, me and Eddie ain't been too close in recent years.

58

I said, Master of understatement.

He said, What's that?

I said, Never mind.

I leaned against the porch railing, worried it would collapse under my weight. Down the street, two kids who didn't look old enough to drive walked out of a ramshackle liquor store drinking from cans in paper bags and disappeared into the Evergreen Cemetery. Without turning to look at him I asked, Were you paroled or did you serve all your time?

He said, I done served it all. What's it to you?

That he wasn't on parole took away my leverage. I asked whether I could check back with him in a week or so. He said, You do that. What was your name again?

■ ■ ■

nstead of driving home I went to the Rothko Chapel. It was nearly six o'clock. One other person was there, a woman who looked to be in her thirties wearing a bright red and purple ankle-length skirt, with beads braided in to her cornrowed hair. She walked over and shook my hand. I must have looked confused. She reminded me she was the sister of a man I had represented. She worked at the Menil Museum bookstore, across the street. I asked her how she was doing, and she said, Plowing on, sir. I am plowing on. She walked quietly out and I sat down on the floor, my back against the rear wall, and looked from one painting to the next.

From the first time I saw the giant canvases, they soothed me. Before I knew Katya, I would come here after every execution. Somehow, the woman at the desk figured out my routine, and when I would arrive, she would say, I'm sorry. Welcome to you, and peace.

I would nod and say thank you and walk into the spare space where quiet pressed into my head. Last year my brother's friend Byron taught me how to look at the paintings. I see more now. I see layers of color, and spaces between the layers. If I can relax my eyes, I see a translucence, almost like the canvases are backlit. My eyes linger longer now on one canvas before they move to the next. Here I am a stick of butter on the beach. I get up to leave and an hour has passed.

There are things you don't perceive because you don't know to look for them, but that doesn't mean they don't affect you. How can I believe that yet also be certain I am not just a brain in a vat? Every single thing we believe, every single fact we take to be true, is underdetermined by the evidence we cite as its proof. It's not just religious people who have faith. The difference between people is whether their faith makes sense.

Until Katya and I got married, I'd go baptize myself after every execution. I'd put my kayak on my truck and go find some moving water, even if I had to drive all the way to the Cossatot in Arkansas. We were drinking at Bitterman's one night and she asked me why I did that. I said, Because maybe my prison is walking through this world all alone.

She said, It's a great song but a stupid lyric. It's your fate only if you choose it.

I said, By that logic, you choose your fate.

She said, Yep.

When I pulled in to the driveway that night she was just getting home from her studio. I told her about my visit with Waterman's dad and my trip to the Rothko. She said, It's not like he knows anything that can help you anyway.

I know. It's just depressing he doesn't even give a shit.

She said, You have this romantic notion that even people who have never in their lives cared about anyone besides themselves are suddenly going to change just because they had unprotected sex.

I said, Doesn't the fact I think it prove it's not romantic?

She said, You might need to make some adjustments to your self-image, cowboy.

■ ■ ■

61

You once told me the problem with generic advice is it ignores individuality. You were criticizing lawyers who make cookie-cutter decisions, indifferent to the particular needs or desires of their clients. Perhaps oncologists are vulnerable to that same critique, because all us cancer patients are the same to them. They are all about the physical. They see the cells but not the person. They do not care about the spirit. They know that to me and everyone else they treat, food has no taste. Colors are dull. Decaying leaves have no smell. But this holds no interest for them.

I probably should not have agreed to have more chemo following the surgery. Every hour I spend connected to an IV feels like a day spent chained to a dungeon wall. I am wasting my little time, and wasting is exactly the right word.

I cannot understand the words on the pages I read. The doctors know this, but it is unimportant to them, because it marks the transition from physical to emotional pain. I suspect they believe this distinction is nonexistent, that all pain has to do with neural pathways, but they are mistaken. There is a difference between debilitating sadness and crushing out a lit cigarette on your thigh.

The physical pain is not my problem. Treating it is therefore not the solution. The problem is the emotional change the physical pain has caused, and it is too late to do anything about that change.

Dr. Nuland says when death is far away, people approach it realistically. They buy insurance. They sign living wills. They execute DNR orders. They plan their funerals. Yet when death is near, they waver. Psychologically, what generates this waver is a denial of death's very proximity. I do not want that to happen, either to me or to those I love. Denial can cause one to pursue futility. Futile pursuits can give false hope. False hope leads to irrational conduct. If it is time, it is time.

My dilemma is that I do not know if it is time, and the people who know I do not trust. Of the two doctors on my team, one is Pollyanna and one is Chicken Little. What I need is a computer. It would lack bedside manner, but it would be entirely free of artifice. I should like to make that exchange.

Irmi and I are going to the Alley Theater on Friday. Will you and Katya join us at Ninfa's beforehand for dinner?

■ ■ ■

On the way to Ninfa's I parked in front of the Char Bar on Travis. Maybe there is such a place in another city besides Houston. It holds a tailor by day and a bar come night. Katya said, You're going to get your one suit altered?

I said, Hah-hah. Actually, I need a drink before I witness the fireworks between you and your dad.

She said, Nope. I am going to be on my best behavior. I am officially giving up on giving advice.

And she was. Peter was going on long walks twice a day. Irmi said he was eating more than he had in months, and his cheeks were less sunken than they had been just two weeks earlier. He was listening to music. I said, Mind over matter.

He said, *I don't think so. I feel cleaner inside. The melanoma might be gone. It might have been limited to the liver after all. The chemicals killed what remained.* Irmi smiled and leaned into him. Katya took a long swallow from her margarita. We ate platters of fajitas and shrimp. Peter ordered honey-drenched sopapillas for dessert. He was so upbeat he seemed drugged. When we got up to leave and told him good night, he said, *Yes, truly it is.*

Katya and I walked to the car with our arms around each other. I knew what she was thinking. She was thinking there was no way

64

he could feel the absence of cancer. She was thinking about the statistics. She was thinking that he knew the statistics. She said, I don't buy it. He's more analytical than you. I don't know whether he's lying to himself or to us. If it's to himself, that's fine. Maybe it means he's decided he wants to live longer. But if it's to us, there's another motivation.

I said, Like maybe he's decided not to do any more chemo?

She said, That's what I'm thinking.

We drove to Ovations and listened to our neighbor's jazz quartet play Thelonius Monk tunes. Between sets, when the lights came up, we saw the conductor and three members of Katya's band. They came over and said hello. When the music started again, Katya said, Can we go home? I don't feel like being in a room with people I know.

■ ■ ■

Waterman had written saying he needed to see me. The guards brought him out right away, but Waterman wasn't smiling. I thought I heard one of them thank him. I said, What was that about?

He said, Aw, nothin' really. They got me living next door to Fierro now. Brother's crazy. Teams got to gas him to get him to the shower. Got a beard like Rasputin.

I said, Rasputin?

He said, I seen pictures. I was talking to him yesterday while they was helmeting up. Just talked him on down, man. Brother's just wound tight, know what I'm sayin'? Anyway, that's all it was.

I asked him how many times he'd talked an inmate into not resisting the guards. He said, Ain't kept count. I guess a few.

I asked him why he needed to see me. His eyes would not meet mine. There were beads of sweat on his forehead. His right knee was bouncing up and down. He said, Dude next door's been teaching me 'bout the Dalai Lama, know who that is? I said I did. He said, So I been thinking the only reason to stay alive is for my daughter, but seeing as she don't want to have nothin' to do with me, ain't no point in staying alive. You see where I'm goin' here?

I said, I think so, but giving up your appeals is not easy. There has to be a hearing. Your case is so far along, I think we should wait to see what happens before you decide to pull the plug. If you're dead, your chance of connecting with your daughter is zero.

He said, Ain't what the Dalai Lama says. Says you can divide the world into people who are good to other people, and those who ain't. Got to try to stay in that first group.

I said, I doubt the Dalai Lama said that.

He said, Don't matter. You remember what you told me? I said I did even though I had no idea what he was referring to. He unbuttoned his jumpsuit to the middle of his chest, reached in, and took out an envelope. He said, You tole me you could send this. He turned the envelope around so I could see the address. He pulled out a single sheet of lined paper and held it up to the glass. It was addressed to Lucy McClain's only surviving relative. The handwriting resembled Lincoln's but the spelling and punctuation were perfect. Waterman had written an apology. He said he used to be in the second group and there was nothing he could do to make up for it, but he wanted the man to know he wasn't in that group anymore. He said, If I was him, I wouldn't forgive me. I ain't asking him to. I just want him to know how I feel, know what I mean? I nodded for him to put the sheet back in the envelope. His eyes were wet.

I said, We'll continue the conversation about giving up your appeals some other time, okay?

He said, All right.

He touched his hand to the glass, then he turned around.

▧　▧　▧

eter taught me to windsurf off the Texas City dike four months
before Katya and I got married. His patience in the face of my
ineptitude was biblical. I fell so frequently my legs were quivering and my hands were raw. After four hours, I managed to tack and sail a rectangle back to where I had started from. Standing hip deep in the channel, Peter raised his arms over his head and applauded. He said, *Bravo, bravo. Now let's eat.*

Irmi had made roast beef sandwiches on sourdough Peter baked the previous night using a starter he had nourished since moving from Oakland more than twenty years before. He said, *You did well, but you're still trying to muscle the board. You're not going to outwrestle the wind. For the big problems, brute strength doesn't work. You'll need finesse.* He opened the Igloo in the back of his Explorer and pulled out a liter of water, a quart of Gatorade, and a bottle of champagne. We sat and drank and watched the sun drop slowly into Galveston Bay.

Peter drove back to their house on the lake. Philip had gotten the weekend off from his job as a computer security specialist and had flown in to visit his parents. Katya and I were spending the weekend in Galveston. At the foot of the causeway I bought a pint of shrimp and a bucket of crabs from two skinny barefoot kids selling seafood and tomatoes from the trunk of their car. Katya and Winona were already at the house. She said, Feel like a short walk while the coals burn down? Winona heard the word *walk*, trotted off to the kitchen, and came back carrying her collar.

We headed toward Sea Isle and watched Saturn climb in the eastern sky. To our right a band of blue floated above the western horizon. Winona chased whitecaps as the tide rolled in. She said, Papa said you did great today.

I said, Either he's lying or you are, but it was fun.

Katya had learned to windsurf nearly before she could swim. She said, Why don't we go to Mexico for our honeymoon? I'm not as good a teacher as Papa, but you have so much to learn it won't matter.

She smiled when she said it. Plus it was true. I said, Hardy har har, and draped my arm across her shoulders. Winona ran over and rammed herself between us.

I called the travel agent the next morning. She said, Are you sure? It's hurricane season in the Caribbean in September. Nobody goes to the Gulf Coast of Mexico. I told her our minds were made up. She said, Well, at least you won't have any trouble getting a honeymoon suite at the finest hotel.

From nearly the beginning of my relationship with Katya, Irmi was wary. I was older, set in my ways, solitary, bookish, and seemingly incapable of compromise. In other words, I lacked every quality a good marriage requires. Plus which culturally speaking, Katya and I were close to opposites, and Irmi thinks platitudes like *opposites attract* are absurd. She said, Katya, I know he adores you, but that's not enough.

One night Katya and I had dinner with my four brothers and their wives at my maternal grandmother's house. My bubbe was born in a Szczuczyn, a Polish village like something out of *Fiddler on the Roof.* Her given name was Rachel. She met her husband, Leon, in Mexico. He and his two brothers had fled Soviet-controlled Lithuania in the 1920s. My Zaide Liebe went to Monterrey. Bubbe worked her way from Poland to Germany and sailed to Mexico because that's where her older brother had gone. Zaide Liebe heard about her from other European refugees. He stood outside her house until she noticed him. That, at least, is the version my aunt tells.

They had my mom in Monterrey, then moved to Nuevo Laredo and started a fabric business. After they moved across the border to Laredo, Texas, Zaide Liebe served as the local rabbi and ran the business until he had a heart attack. Bubbe took over. This was the 1940s. Alone, she would travel from Laredo to New York to buy and back to Texas and Mexico to sell.

Bubbe spoke eight languages, made homemade gefilte fish, smoked Carltons down to the filter, went to synagogue three times a week, played high-stakes poker in Vegas, and loved raunchy jokes. That night at dinner she told one: *A woman is standing outside but there isn't a minyan. Nine men are inside. They need a tenth for a service. The elderly woman sees a Jewish man walking by and says to him, Excuse me please, sir. But will you come inside? You'll be the tenth.* Bubbe told it in English until she got to the punch line. Then she said, *Der Mann schaute sie von oben bis unten an und sagte, Gnädige Frau, ich würde es nicht tun, selbst wenn ich der erste wäre.*

Bubbe crossed her hands over her mouth and guffawed like a stevedore. Katya laughed too. She looked at me and I shrugged. My mother's first language was Spanish, which she taught to her sons. But when it comes to Yiddish, her second tongue, my brothers and I speak hardly a word. Yiddish is mostly German, though, and German was Katya's first language. So Katya said, It means the man looked her up and down and said, Madam, I wouldn't do it even if I were the first.

My brother Steven and his wife Stacy turned red. My brother Mark said, Wow. My bubbe pulled Katya toward her and kissed her on the head.

I told Peter the story the next day. He said, *Irmi will say that the same sentiment that caused your grandmother to hug Katya last night will make her distrustful in a week. History is more powerful than sentimentality.*

I said, You don't really believe that.

He said, *I'm not talking about me.*

I have no proof that Peter actually lobbied Irmi on my behalf. When I asked him that day in Texas City, he smiled and said, *As you'll soon learn, we husbands have to keep some things secret.*

It doesn't matter. I know he was on my side. And one thing I've learned is that moral support matters for reasons reason cannot fully explain. It's why death row inmates ask their lawyers to witness their executions. It's why misery loves company and the best thing you can do for your friend at his mother's funeral is to hug him and say not a word. That Peter knew I would be good for his daughter made me sure I would be.

To say thanks, Katya and I invited him to go to North Carolina with us two weeks before our wedding. I'd kayak on the Ocoee and Chattooga during the day while Katya and Peter would hike in the Smoky Mountains. At night, we'd cook dinner at our cabin, drink cheap champagne, listen to the creek, and watch the stars. That was the plan.

The first day, my paddling buddy Dave and I were running a steep technical drop on Indian Creek. We scouted it from river right. The best line was left to right. We were going to ferry across and spin into the rapid from the opposite side. You ferry by pointing your boat upstream and angling the bow in the direction you want to go. The speed of the current dictates the degree of your angle. Paddling out of the eddy, mine wasn't adequately oblique. The current spun me clockwise 270 degrees and into the rapid backward. I ping-ponged off a rock on the right side of the riverbank and went over the drop perpendicular to the current. My stern caromed off a rock behind me I never saw, and I flipped. The 50-degree water tightened my chest. I missed my roll. I was recirculating in the hole we had picked our line to avoid. Upside down in the water, I reached down with my paddle and felt myself wash free. I set up to roll again. I twisted at the waist and reached up with my hands to feel the air, but the downstream side of my boat was pinned against a rock. I went to set up to roll on my other side and missed again. I did not want to have to swim in this water. The boiling rapid was a quarter mile long. I set up once more. A good Eskimo roll is all hip action and head. You don't need the paddle. But I was low on oxygen and cold and starting to panic, and when I flicked my hip and my head, I also drove my right arm down hard. I felt the water's resistance to the paddle blade, and then a pain like a red-hot knife was prying my arm from my shoulder. I came up with such velocity I almost flipped over the opposite direction. I paddled one-armed to an eddy where Dave was setting up to throw me a rope.

In Bryson City, the emergency room doctor popped my dislocated shoulder back in place and told me the MRI showed three torn tendons in my right rotator cuff. He wrote a prescription for painkillers. I drank two bottles of beer at the Rite Aid while I waited on it to be filled.

At our cabin I washed down two pills with a tall glass of bourbon and shaved ice, and by sunset I was feeling grand. Peter and I dredged fresh trout in cornmeal and fried them in a cast-iron skillet while Katya tossed a salad and heated pinto beans from a can. Years later, shortly after Lincoln was born, my memory of that day would be one of the reasons I gave whitewater up, but that night I told them I intended to run the same drop tomorrow. Back in the saddle, I said, drunk and teeming with Texas clichés. Instead, I spent most of the next day unconscious, my right arm useless, while Katya and Peter hiked the Appalachian Trail. We flew back to Houston three days ahead of schedule.

Windsurfing was out of the question. The travel agent sounded relieved when I called her. She found us a room at a resort in the Rockies where we could go hiking from our back door.

As it happens, 1996 was the busiest year on record for Atlantic hurricanes. The week leading up to our marriage, hurricanes Cesar and Dolly killed nearly seventy people in Mexico and Central America. The week of our wedding, Hurricane Eduard formed, with winds of more than 145 miles per hour. While Katya and I were climbing Pike's Peak, Hurricane Hortense was pummeling Puerto Rico and the U.S. Virgin Islands.

We stopped for lunch at the spot where Katharine Lee Bates supposedly wrote *America the Beautiful* in 1893. Katya is the opposite of her mom. She believes the sheer improbability of our finding each other is proof we belong together. She said, If you hadn't hurt yourself, we'd probably be sitting somewhere in the Yucatán with no power. We would never have come to this amazing spot. You think that was a mere coincidence?

He's wrong, of course, but I know what Blake meant when he

said science robs us of our spirit. Any time you do the math, wonder gives way to ennui. Everything that happens makes perfect sense.

Still, I put my good arm around my wife's shoulders and pulled her toward me. I kissed her ear and I said, Maybe not.

■ ■ ■

L incoln wanted to go out to the field behind our house and play Frisbee with Winona. I said, Okay, but let's work a little first.

Lincoln was on my right. He was still at the age when he would let me hold his hand. Winona walked on our left, slightly in front of us, leading the way. I said, *Left*, and she turned left. We walked a football-field-size rectangle, speeding up and slowing down, then I put her in an off-leash heel, with her nose behind my knee, and we walked tight figure-eights. I said, *Up*, and she looked up, then *Back*, and she turned around. Lincoln was bored and anxious to play. I put Winona in a down-stay, and Lincoln and I walked back toward the house.

He said, Dada, why do you keep doing things with Winona she already knows how to do?

I said, Because, Linco, you play like you practice.

He said, That makes sense.

I said, Go ahead and call her now.

Lincoln said, Nonie, come. She rocketed over and lay down at his feet. Lincoln put the Frisbee on her head like a hat. He grabbed her ears and kissed her nose.

I trained Winona using the modified Koehler method (invented by Bill Koehler, modified by me). The first step in the Koehler method is to condition the dog to be focused on the handler all the time. This is not a Zen approach to dog training. When you are teaching an eight-month-old dog to be focused on you no matter what happens, no matter whether a cat or a squirrel or a T-bone steak crosses her path, physicality is at times required. I would correct her by pinching her ear.

My dog Whitney, Winona's predecessor, almost died when she got hit by a car lunging after a feral cat. A kind passerby who drove us to the clinic, a quick-thinking vet, two blood transfusions, and a helping of luck saved her life. Sometimes nobody is at fault. Sometimes someone is. Now I train my dogs to save their lives. That they are also better pets is just the gilding.

But anyone can train a robot. You also want your dog to think.

Shopping for dinner is when I like to get lost in my thoughts, so I trained Winona to get us to the store. If I say *Whole Foods, sidewalk*, she knows to lead us to Whole Foods on the sidewalk, which is a different command from *Whole Foods, street*. If there is a pile of leaves on the sidewalk, she walks us straight through them. But if there is a broken tree limb dangling in my path, or a deep puddle left over from last night's rain, Winona will stop and get my attention. She knows we should leave the sidewalk so I can stay dry and scratch-free, despite my earlier command.

When Winona was two she adopted a cat. A week-old abandoned kitten found her way to our Galveston house. Katya named her Mazel, which means luck. Winona would carry Mazel in her mouth and use her front teeth to pick nits from the kitten's fur. They ate their meals together and drank from the same bowl. The cat would bang on the door when she needed to go out, and bang again when ready to come back in. When we took our nightly stroll, Mazel walked with us in Winona's shadow. She slept curled in a U under Winona's snout.

While Lincoln was kissing Winona's nose, Mazel walked over and sat down like a spectator. Lincoln kneeled down and stroked her head. He said, Dada, can we please play Frisbee now? He threw the disc pretty well for a seven-year-old kid. Winona brought it back to him and dropped it at his feet. Lincoln said, Now Nonie's happy.

■　■　■

I was not lying to you at Ninfa's, but I am now convinced I was wrong. I can feel the cancer. It is a sludge in my brain. When Philip was here, he told me about a problem he had solved. He and I are both scientists, in a manner of speaking, yet I could scarcely follow him. He made me feel obsolete. Let me put it to you this way: I do not understand music I used to love.

Peter was referring to a story I told him in North Carolina about the first time I heard the studio recording of "Ko Ko." Charlie Parker on sax, Max Roach playing drums, Bud Powell at the piano, and Miles Davis on trumpet. Dizzy Gillespie was there just to watch. But Powell didn't show, because he had gotten arrested the night before and was still in jail, so Dizzy would be on keyboard. They start to play and—this is almost impossible to believe, but you have to re-member that Miles was only nineteen at the time—Davis could not keep up. So Dizzy played piano and trumpet. He and Parker start off with fairly typical call and answer, then Roach comes in, bang, and Parker takes off. He's playing so fast you can't hear the melody. At least I couldn't. This was back in the Sony Walkman days, when you could control the tape speed. I slowed it as far as it would go and it was magic. The melody formed, like when you are staring at those nonsense paintings and suddenly there's a three-dimensional image. I gradually sped it back to normal, and I could still hear it. I had said to Peter, It shattered my belief that beauty is universal, and therefore that anything is universal, and that makes me sad.

He said, *It shouldn't, not at all. Hable mas depacio, por favor. I've heard you say that when you are talking to Mexicans who speak like machine guns. You know the words but you can't hear them. Music and language are no different.* I looked unconvinced. He said, *That your brain must learn truths does not mean there are no truths.*

Now he wrote, *I know what is happening to me, or what used to be me. You remember what I told you about "Ko Ko"? Your brain processes faster as it learns. This is a unidirectional process, because it is impossible to unlearn something you know. What that means, therefore, is that if you start to process more slowly, it can only be because your brain is dying.*

Last night I was listening to Glenn Gould's radical recording of the Goldberg Variations. *From the first time I heard this recording thirty years ago, it moved me deeply. It was perfect in every way. Last night, it was too fast. It was too fast, and I did not understand.*

I need you to help me. I know you know how to let go. Did you have to learn how to tell a man he would be dead in thirty minutes because the appeal was denied, or did this come naturally to you? It doesn't matter. I need you to teach it to Katya. Thankfully I can still tell from moments like last night that I am changing, but this too will not last. Soon I will not know myself and nor will I be myself, and I will not know I do not know. It will be better for me, and better for Katya, if she winds down with me.

How is it going for your gangster?

■ ■ ■

We won our case in the federal district court. After a weeklong hearing at which two pathologists and the trial lawyer took the witness stand, the judge concluded it was probable that Miss McClain was already dead when Waterman shot her and that, if the jury had known that fact, it might not have sentenced him to death. He was entitled to a new trial. Cara and Jeffrey wanted to go out and celebrate and toast my decision to focus on a winning issue, but I knew better. I told them I had plans but they should have a beer or two on my tab, and I watched as they glided over to O'Neill's, convinced they had saved a life.

When I went to the prison to tell Waterman the next day, he said, How come you don't seem all that excited? This is good news, ain't it? I told him the problem was that the attorney general's office planned to appeal, and it would be hard for us to hold on to our victory. He said, Even if I agree to a life sentence they're gonna appeal to try to kill me anyway? I told him they were. He said, Shit. I been here ten years. No matter how much you change who you are, you cain't change what you done. He hung up the phone without telling me good-bye and turned his back. As I was standing up to leave he turned back around. He mouthed, I'm sorry, and he touched his hand to the glass.

My colleagues in the history department might expel me from the ivory tower for saying this, but you know that aphorism about how people who forget history are condemned to repeat it? Well, I think Santayana had it backward. People who remember the past can't escape it. Listen to Israelis and Palestinians argue about peace, or Greeks and Turks fight over Cyprus, or two siblings carp about anything, and it's all about who started it. It's a contest to see who can document the earliest historical grievance and then use that episode to justify everything that follows, like steps in a syllogism. History isn't a lesson. It's a leash. Forgetting, on the other hand, frees you to start over.

I was busy trying to forget about Samuel Norton the night before I flew to New Orleans to argue Waterman's case before the federal court of appeals. Norton would be one of the three judges to rule on the appeal. Here's what I was trying not to remember: Years ago there was a death row inmate named Calvin Burdine. A federal judge ruled he was entitled to a new trial because his trial lawyer had repeatedly fallen asleep during the trial. When the case got to the court of appeals, Samuel Norton, along with one other judge, voted to reverse the trial judge and reinstate the conviction and death sentence. (The third judge on the panel dissented, agreeing with the lower court judge that Burdine deserved a new trial.) The entire court of appeals elected to rehear the case and, by a vote of nine to five, upheld the decision of the lower court. I was trying to forget there were five appellate court judges who believed it was perfectly okay to execute someone whose trial lawyer had slept through the proceedings and that one of those five would be the senior judge hearing Waterman's case.

I tell my students there's a difference between law and ideology, but the difference vanishes when the judges are ideologues, and

Judge Norton is the proof. Here's part of the gauzy justification he offered up in defense of his belief that the State of Texas should be permitted to execute Burdine after providing him a somnambulant lawyer. He said it was not clear *When [the lawyer] "dozed" as opposed to "slept."* He wondered *How long he slept* and *How many times he slept* and *How deeply he slept.* He asked *When the sleeping occurred— which day(s), or whether during the morning or afternoon.* Nine judges, of course, thought these questions were idiotic, but they were not the judges who would be deciding my case. Norton thought his colleagues were overburdening lower court judges. He complained that the ruling on behalf of Burdine was going to *impose . . . a new obligation on the States . . . by requiring trial judges . . . to closely and unceasingly monitor defense counsel throughout trial to ensure defense counsel is awake.*

Three other judges agreed with Norton's so-called analysis. I was trying to forget about them, too. One of them was also going to be hearing Waterman's appeal.

Judging the winner of a legal argument is more like judging a gymnastics competition than a 100-meter dash. If a Russian and an American are running against each other, the nationality of the person who fires the starter's pistol is irrelevant. But if they're competing against each other on the balance beam, it's a different story. Representing death row inmates from Texas in front of the federal court of appeals for the Fifth Circuit in New Orleans is like being an American gymnast competing against Olga Korbut in Moscow before three judges who work for the Kremlin. You're there to jump through the hoops and for your pride, because there is almost no chance you're going to win. People who think bogus legal proceedings happen only in places like Iran or China apparently haven't been to Texas.

It hasn't always been this way. Dyed-in-the-wool conservative jurists appointed by conservative presidents brought the end of racial segregation to the South. But decent judges have been replaced by bureaucratic hacks who reach results that melt their political butter no matter how much violence they have to inflict on legal principles on the way to getting there. Samuel Norton would make two plus two equal six if that's what it took to uphold a death sentence of a convicted murderer. Waterman's lawyer had made some serious mistakes, but he had been awake when he made them, and that meant he cleared the bar Norton had set in the *Burdine* case.

Waterman didn't have a chance.

After the argument, during which Norton might as well have been wearing an executioner's hood, a reporter who had been in the courtroom came up to me and asked what exactly had gone on. I said, I've always found it fitting that the first known use of the expression *kangaroo court* appeared in a nineteenth-century magazine article called *A Stray Yankee in Texas*. The reporter asked whether my comment was on the record. I said, Of course. The only question here is whether this panel of quote judges unquote will already have ruled against us by the time I get back to Texas.

What defenders of Santayana's dictum might say in his defense is that forgetting is not all that different from sticking your head in the sand. History does repeat itself, and you can't change the facts by ignoring them. They do have a point. Still, Norton and his colleagues surprised me. It took them nearly three months to issue the opinion reversing the lower court's ruling.

◼ ◼ ◼

MIDDLES

y solo un hombre soy de carne y hueso,
por eso si apalean a mi hermano
con lo que tengo a mano lo defiendo.
           —Pablo Neruda, "No Me Lo Pidan"

igh school English is where I first learned not everybody can be understood by everyone. It's in *As I Lay Dying,* chapter 19. Vardaman says, My mother is a fish.

That's it. End of chapter. My teacher wanted to tell us what Faulkner meant. I didn't feel the need to know. You can like a rhythm or savor a sound, and not have a clue what it means.

Not knowing is itself knowledge. At the beginning I think I can learn. At the end I know I cannot. It is the middle where I see the truth.

Perhaps it is merely fortuitous that Vardaman's soliloquy begins the middle third of Faulkner's book.

The deepest knowledge, I've learned, can be awareness of the chasm separating you from someone else.

■ ■ ■

During the first three years of Lincoln's life, I would take him running with me. Winona trotted along on the left side of the jogging stroller. One morning our neighbor Linda walked over to see how Lincoln was doing. When she peered down into the stroller, Winona growled. The leash stayed slack. Winona was just letting her know she was watching.

People think Dobermans are inherently vicious. It's not true. They're like people. How they act is a direct function of how they're raised. Winona came with me to the office every day and slept in our bed at night. She sensed when people feared her and took steps to allay their concerns. If burglars had ever entered our house, Winona would have lifted her head from the sofa and watched them as they carted out our furniture, our music, our piano, every volume in our library. But if Lincoln had been asleep on the second floor, and they'd set even one foot on the stairs, Winona would have cleaved their throats.

Lincoln called me at the office to say Winona was worse. Ever since our Frisbee session she had been walking gingerly, but at least she would walk. Each evening at dusk, after Lincoln's piano practice, Winona would take her leash in her mouth and stand at the back door, waiting for us. But on that day, when Lincoln finished playing and called to her, she only raised her head. She made no move to stand.

Katya made an appointment at the vet to see if there was anything we could do for her arthritis. Lincoln asked me to come home early to take her.

When I got home twenty minutes later, Lincoln was waiting for me in the kitchen, eating. He waved at me with a spoon. He used his index finger to put some of the ice cream onto a second spoon and fed it to Winona. He said, Is it time to go?

I said, Yes it is, Linco. And stop feeding Winona.

He said, Mama does it.

I said, Ice cream?

He said, No, but other things. Why does that matter?

The three of us drove to the vet. The vet said, There's a new drug for dogs called Metacam. You should see improvement by this weekend.

Lincoln said, By this weekend? You do realize today is already Thursday?

The vet looked at me and smiled. She turned back to Lincoln. She said, Yes, I do realize that. The drug works very rapidly.

Lincoln said, Okay then.

When we got home we gave her the first dose. Three hours later Winona hopped onto the sofa. It was the first time she'd done that in three weeks. Lincoln and I were in the kitchen boiling pasta. Lincoln said, Wow. That was even faster than I was expecting.

■ ■ ■

Metacam is a nonsteroidal anti-inflammatory (or NSAID). It works by blocking the production of prostaglandins. It does that by interfering with cyclooxygenase, or COX, an enzyme needed to produce prostaglandin in the tissue. Prostaglandins are a family of chemicals that, among other things, makes us sensitive to pain. Winona had the same arthritis at seven o'clock that she had at three, but her pain was no longer debilitating.

To know whether it makes sense to trade quantity for quality, you have to run the numbers. Peter was refusing more chemotherapy because he opted for six good months over eighteen inferior ones. Maybe he was undervaluing the benefit of the additional year, but at least he did the math.

We made the choice for Winona without knowing we were making it. The prostaglandins the Metacam was suppressing also regulate blood flow to the kidneys and protect the stomach's lining. So she—we—were risking her kidneys in exchange for less joint pain. Is it possible for a choice to be the right one if you don't know it's a choice?

Here are a few other things we didn't know: NSAIDs can cause ulceration and bleeding in the gastrointestinal tract. They can trigger kidney failure. They can do permanent liver damage, and it can be life threatening. There was a lot to watch out for, if you knew to watch out.

Waterman had written me a letter about Donald Starret. They were neighbors. Starret had asked Waterman to ask me if I would make sure nobody tried to intervene in his case. Starret had fired his lawyer and told the federal judge presiding over his case he wanted to give up his appeals and be executed as soon as possible. The court obliged and set his execution for January 8. In death penalty argot, he was a volunteer. As I've said, a death row inmate who forfeits his appeals because he would rather be executed soon than spend years on death row might well be making a rational choice. Of course, I didn't know whether Starret actually had the capacity to reason, but I was worrying about too many other dying beings to care. I wrote him and said I couldn't help. He wrote me back, said he had five thousand dollars and wanted to hire me.

I was confused, too. Unless they are mentally impaired, inmates are permitted to fire their lawyers and waive their appeals. They write the judge, the judge holds a hearing, usually listening to testimony from the inmate, the inmate's lawyer, and a psychologist or two, then makes a decision. I called the lawyer Starret had fired to let him know Starret had written me. He said, Sure, go see the guy. He's as sane as you or me. He wants to ride the needle now 'stead of being some dude's wife for five years, makes sense to me. Believe me, I tried to talk him out of it, but the guy's mind is made up.

Maybe the lawyer was being metaphorical. Death row inmates have no physical contact with other inmates. Or maybe he's just an ass. Either way, I asked Cara to conduct an intake interview.

When new prisoners arrive at death row, one of the lawyers who works with me conducts an initial interview. It can last two full days.

We try to learn every school, hospital, jail, prison, mental institution, and city where the person has ever been. We want to know every member of his family, going back three generations, and every teacher, friend, and parole officer he's ever had. A good death penalty lawyer knows more about her client than she knows about her spouse, maybe than she knows about herself. I didn't think we'd find any Nobel laureates in Starret's family tree. I was interested in the opposite phenomenon. Mental illness runs in families just like heart disease does. If your dad dropped dead of a heart attack at age fifty, you watch your cholesterol and take certain medicine as a precaution. Just because Starret's relatives might have been in mental institutions didn't mean his decision to volunteer wasn't rational. It just meant there was something I should know about.

When Starret walked into the booth I got my first impression. His nails were clean and trimmed. His hair was short. His teeth, though, while white as bone, looked like pieces of a jigsaw puzzle. He wasn't lying when he told Cara he'd done a lot of crystal meth. I made a note to see how much he'd smoked the day he did his crime.

In prison there are two kinds of crazy people. Some you recognize as crazy in thirty seconds. Others you can talk to for five hours and not realize they're three cards shy until fifteen minutes before you go home. I spent two hours with Starret and concluded he fell into neither category. We talked about his crime (he killed his girlfriend's mother), his lawyers (not the best, not the worst), his prospects for getting off death row (exceedingly remote), how long his appeals would take (four years minimum, seven years max), and whether conditions on death row would improve significantly in the near term (not a chance). He said, I just don't want to live like this. You feel me?

I said nothing and just looked at him. He ran his tongue back and forth across his upper teeth like a windshield wiper.

I asked whether there was anything I could do for him. He said, I ain't seen my mother or daughter since I been here. You think you could get them to come see me? I said I'd try.

On the drive home I called Cara. I said, The guy's totally normal. Let's get a transcript of the competency hearing to make sure the court dotted all the i's, but I don't think we'll be getting involved. Can you just do me a favor and track down his mom and daughter and see what it will take to get them to go visit?

Cara said, What are you talking about?

I said, He asked me to see if I could get his mom and daughter to visit before the execution.

Cara said, His mom died two years ago. His daughter was there with him yesterday for two hours before I interrupted them.

I said, Oops.

■　■　■

That night Peter called to say the oncologist wanted him to undergo one more round of chemotherapy. Peter said, *He told me it is the accepted protocol. I said, Accepted by whom? He said, Melanoma specialists. I asked him how much longer I would live with it than without. He said he could not be sure. I told him it is hard to make a decision with no data.*

Peter said, *What I did not say to him is that following a course of therapy simply because everyone follows it is not science. It is a way to pretend to care.*

He asked me how the argument in the court of appeals had gone. I said, I had a fried shrimp po' boy and a bowl of gumbo at Mother's, and I paid for the trip by playing poker at Harrah's. Besides the food and the cards, the trip was a waste of a beautiful day. I could have helped Waterman as much by taking a walk along the Mississippi.

He listened to my report. He said, *Some mediocre men are ambitious, and their mediocrity thwarts them. As a consequence, they become angry. Angry people feel they are failures, and they lash out at others. Don't you remember* American Slavery, American Freedom? *You ought not to blame yourself for not getting through to him. His hostility to your client arises from how he feels about himself.*

I laughed and said, Since when did you become an armchair psychologist?

He said, *I am reading* Crime and Punishment, *or trying to. Dostoevsky is a better teacher of psychology than a college textbook.*

I said, Well, nearly all the judges on the court of appeals think they belong on the Supreme Court. If my only hope of saving Waterman is to find a few who are happy with their lots, Waterman is in dire straits.

Peter said, *At least the man who is trying to save his life knows the numbers.*

■ ■ ■

On my second day of third grade, I got home from school and was greeted by a woman named Evelina. My mom had hired her as a housekeeper that morning. Evelina was six foot five and weighed 260. Her skin was the color of ink. She took my lunch box from me and said, Hi. I'm Evelina, Evelina Dow. I have the same last name as you do. You know what that means? She paused for me to answer, but I just stood and stared. So Evelina filled the silence. She always filled the silence. She said, It means we're related.

She smiled and I could see gold crowns on half her teeth. I looked down at her feet. She had cut off the ends of her sneakers to make room for her diabetically swollen toes. I stalled. When would my mother be home? I finally said, I don't think so, Evelina.

Her eyes sparkled. She was the first practical joker I had met. She said, It doesn't? Why not?

I stammered for a while, then I said, Well, you see, Evelina, we're Jewish.

I don't actually remember that happening, but Evelina told the story a hundred times. When she repeated what I supposedly said, she tilted her head back and clapped her hands and the laugh that started in her substantial belly was a sound of pure joy.

Evelina would wrap her mammoth arms around my brothers and me when we behaved, and chase us out of the house with a broom when we did not. She taught me how to cook chicken and dumplings and make biscuits from scratch. She invented fried chicken and hush puppies. When I rode with her in her Dodge Dart to the grocery store, I felt as safe as when I was with my dad.

Evelina's son had run in George Foreman's gang in the '60s. Evelina told me Foreman used to eat in her kitchen when he was still a delinquent. Foreman went to the Olympics, won a gold medal in 1968, became heavyweight champion of the world. Evelina's son died of a heroin overdose.

I moved back to Texas in the late 1980s and started sparring at an inner city gym on a not-yet-gentrified street. I hadn't talked to Evelina in at least ten years. But when the phone rang I recognized her husky voice as soon as she said my name. She said, I talked to your mama. You need to promise me you'll stay away from the Fourth Ward. I didn't answer. She said, Promise me, son.

Two weeks later I was sitting next to my mom in the church at Evelina's funeral. Evelina had not worked for my family for many years, but my mom still gave her money to pay the electric bill. After the eulogy, the preacher walked up to my mother and thanked her for supporting the church. Evelina, we learned, had been giving her electricity money to the Sunday collection plate. There are people who disguise the rudiments of their goodness all the way to the grave, but no one can hide who she really is.

One of my clients is possibly the smartest man in prison. I'm not just referring to the inmates. He graduated from college with a degree in civil engineering, speaks four languages, and reads a thousand pages a week of novels, poetry, science, and architecture. On nights following days when I've seen him, I dream of wasted lives. He once asked me whether it wasn't highly inefficient for me to spend a day driving to and from the prison just to say things to a client I could easily put in a letter. I smiled. I said, From a purely economic point of view, yes it is. He sent a letter thanking me for the visit and included an algorithm for how he thought I should spend my time.

Some death penalty lawyers criticize other death penalty lawyers for not visiting their clients enough. Some clients think they are being ill served if their lawyer doesn't come to see them weekly. But death row is in the middle of nowhere. It's a two-hour drive from Houston, a four-hour drive from Dallas, a day trip from the valley. Cancer doctors don't stand there chatting with the patient while the IVs are dripping. Once I've conducted a complete intake interview, there is hardly anything I can't learn from a letter.

But there are some guys like Starret whose camouflaged lunacy can hide for years, and others like Waterman whose surprising depth can take days to plumb. I remembered Evelina every time I went to see him. If someone like her had been his mom, I know this for sure, I would never have met him. After the argument in the court of appeals, I had gone to the prison to tell him how badly it had gone. He said, Say what? And when I repeated myself, he did not reply.

He was not a good enough actor to convince me he was listening. I said, What's up?

Waterman's sister Hattie had told him his dad was dying from lung cancer. I didn't think he'd care. Waterman had been in prison more than ten years, and the last contact with his father had been five years before he went in. Waterman's family tree looked like a

Pollock painting, full of step- and half siblings. As best we could figure, his dad had fathered a dozen children by eight women. Waterman's only full brother shot himself in the heart on his tenth birthday because his girlfriend dumped him, and Waterman hardly knew any of the others. I did not have to assume his father was an ass. I'd met him.

If that was your history, can you imagine being sad when your father died? If you can, you might be a little too generous with forgiveness.

He asked whether I'd found a way for him to go to the funeral, and when I told him no tears spilled out of his eyes.

I told him about the details of the argument and what would happen next. He just nodded. He asked whether I could get his daughter to write him. He said, There ain't much I got to teach her, 'cept to tell her to pretty much do the opposite of me. Matter of fact, only reason I got any interest in staying alive is so's I can try to be a little bit of a father 'fore I die.

He was giving up again, and my first thought was that at least it would be easier on me when I had to tell him he was about to die.

All this happened before Jeffrey and Cara had persuaded me the best thing we could do for him was to stress who Waterman had become. I was still focused on explaining how he had gotten to be someone who could do something so bad. The problem with this approach from the death penalty lawyer's standard playbook is that most people, including most judges, tend to equate *explanation* with *excuse*. As soon as you start the story of how a kid grew up with neither a father nor a mother and his only friend, his older brother, killed himself when he was ten, and his mother was psychotic and a crackhead and his father was philandering and violent, and the kid therefore, at age eleven, ended up in a gang because it was literally the only family (lit. *members of a household*) he had, they say, Sure, but that's no excuse. Lots of kids have it tough.

One thing I've learned is that the people who say that never did.

■　■　■

K atya, Lincoln, Winona, and I drove to Galveston for a three-day weekend. As we were crossing the causeway, Jeffrey called. He said, Kathy says they're setting a date for Waterman on Tuesday. Do you want to go to the hearing or should I?

Kathy is an assistant DA. She called us because Texas is different from other death penalty states. Instead of having a central office set all executions, individual district attorneys do it. They plan them around their vacations. Some will coordinate with the inmate's lawyer, if their relationship with him is good. But Kathy didn't call me to work something out. She called with an edict. You might think the judge is the actual person in charge, and strictly speaking you would be right, but the judge was probably a district attorney before she won an election. She is probably married to a prosecutor. She goes on vacation and to happy hour with district attorneys. She routinely does what the prosecutor asks her to do. Anybody who tells you the criminal justice system is an even playing field has no idea what she's talking about. Rich people can make it close to even. Poor people—which is to say, everyone on death row—don't have a chance.

The other special thing about Texas is that the state executes people before their appeals are over. Once an inmate loses in the court of appeals, he has a right to ask the Supreme Court to review the case. He has ninety days to file that request. The Supreme Court's rules require the state to respond to the inmate's request. The state has thirty days to do so. But they typically ask for and get extensions of thirty or sixty days more. Then the Court "conferences" the inmate's petition, meaning the Court decides whether to hear the appeal. All told, that process takes six months to a year. Ninety percent of the time the Court says no. Everywhere except Texas, once the Court turns down the appeal, the state might set the execution date. In Texas, district attorneys set execution dates before the process is completed, before the Supreme Court has said no. Sometimes they set the dates before the inmate's appeal has been filed. We routinely ask the justices to intervene and prevent this practice. It's one thing for them to turn down an inmate's appeal. It's another for them to let an inmate be killed before the paperwork is done. The Great Awakening for law students comes on the day they realize that law, like war, is just an extension of politics, where principle routinely bends before expediency and ideology. Even the so-called liberal justices stand idly by while the state executes people whose appeals are not complete. There are days I'm embarrassed to be a member of the profession.

I told Jeffrey I'd cover it, and I made plans to go tell Waterman he'd be put to death while his appeal lay pending.

We stopped at Seven Seas for groceries. My foul mood clung to me like stink. Lincoln said, Dada, you should also buy some ice cream. It will cheer you up.

I said, I don't want any ice cream, and we are only here for two days. It will go to waste.

He said, No it won't. I'll eat it. Blue Bell Vanilla always pleases me. He took his index fingers and lifted my mouth into the shape of a smile. He said, Feel better now?

I bought steaks, potatoes to mash with garlic and buttermilk, Campari tomatoes for a salad, and of course the ice cream. Lincoln said, Guess how long it takes at the Blue Bell factory to make a pint of ice cream?

I said, I don't know, Linco.

Guess.

I don't know.

Just guess.

Okay. One hour.

No, Dada.

There is a thin tonal line between indulgence and disappointment. I wasn't sure which side I was hearing. I took another guess. Finally Lincoln told me the answer. For the ten minutes it took to drive from the store to our house, nobody said a word.

■　■　■

I was talking to the rabbi about boundaries. Irmi and I are children of Nazism, even if our parents were not Nazis. Everyone who grew up in our time carries that burden. So we tried to raise our children without them. There are not Lutherans and Catholics, we said, just good people and bad people. And the result is that they grew up without a community. Where will they turn for comfort or meaning when we are dead? Did we serve them well or betray them? Is it my fault Katya spends her evenings searching for exotic untested therapies so I might live awhile longer?

I agree with you, as you know, when you say religion is authoritarian, when you insist religious dogma and ideology thereby foster authoritarianism and the surrender of independence. I believe you are correct to say religion reinforces and perhaps even creates the insidious distinction between us and them. I even share your view that raising children in a religious tradition is nothing short of brainwashing.

But perhaps, I said to the rabbi, these boundaries are hard-wired, left over from when membership in a tribe was a key to survival. Our ethical philosophy outruns natural selection, so we are left with ideas that make sense but that are not true. You can imagine a world without boundaries, but it's like a world of five dimensions. It is not our world. If you ask me how something can be both sensible as well as false, I would answer that it resides in the vaporous boundary that separates reality from aspiration. Did Irmi and I raise our children under the spell *of an illusion? It is one thing to aspire to an ideal in one's own life. It is quite another to gamble the well-being of your children on that aspiration.*

Everything important we learn too late. The better parental strategy would have been not to eschew boundaries altogether but to teach that the lines we use to make sense of our world are elusive. Someone who tells a tasteless joke at a dinner party might be a racist, or he might just have bad taste.

The same goes for the line between life and death. For Katya, either I am here or I am not. For me, the line is elusive. If I submit to more chemotherapy and fight, I will die. If I tell the doctor no, I will die. Either way, I will never climb another mountain.

I am certain I appeared to him ingenuous, but still I asked the rabbi, If there is God, why is there painful death? His reply was not an answer.

You are the one who argues volunteers can be rational. Remaining alive is not worth every price. I do not know how to say that to Katya without sounding cruel.

▨ ▨ ▨

It rained for two days. The waves were four feet but too sloppy for the surfing to be any good. I paddled my kayak out past the third sandbar and worked on my Eskimo roll until I was dizzy. Katya, Lincoln, and I played Scrabble, Pictionary, and Blokus. I finished third every time. An hour before we had to drive back to Houston the sun came out. Lincoln said we should take a short walk with Winona before we headed home. I cut the end off a cigar. Lincoln said, You're not going to smoke that, are you?

The first time Winona came to the beach she was six weeks old and weighed eleven pounds. On the western end of the island, the horizon can seem endless and the pounding surf is loud. Winona vibrated like a piano string. I picked her up and carried her for a mile. The next day at dawn she sprinted into the gulf. A wave broke over her head. She shook herself dry and smiled. From that day on, she pranced down the beach like Marmaduke. I believe she thought she owned it.

The four of us headed west, toward Surfside. We watched three herons in a line knife into the surf and surface with mullet hanging from their mouths. Winona usually ran ahead, chasing gulls into the surf before circling back. This day, she lagged far behind, then stopped walking altogether. She would come to me when I called her, but then she would stay where she was until I called her again. When I touched her belly she winced.

Katya said, Can you carry her home? Back at the house I put her on the sofa while we packed up. When Lincoln sat down next to her, she snapped. He put his hand on her hip and started to cry.

We drove straight to the emergency clinic instead of going home. A technician drew blood and asked about her symptoms. The doctor came in and asked what medications she was on. I told him Metacam. He said, For how long? Then he said, Most dogs have no problems with it.

I thought to myself, *Most* can mean *barely* more than half. But Lincoln and Katya were standing there next to me, barely holding it together, so I said nothing. He ordered an abdominal ultrasound, a fecal exam, a urinalysis, and a complete blood test, including a packed cell volume test. I asked what he was looking for. He said, Whether she's bleeding, and whether she has liver failure.

We sat there flipping through old magazines in a windowless fluorescent-lit room that hid the time. From somewhere a dog barked, and I realized I wasn't sure I could tell Winona's bark from another dog's. Before that thought could level me, they brought Winona back out and sent us home. The doctor said, We might have to do a bone marrow aspirate, but I think stopping the medicine should do the trick.

The lab called the following afternoon. Winona's blood work was normal and the other tests were negative. I said, Well then what was the matter?

The lab worker said, The doctor said to tell you that you should get her some Geritol, and you should see improvement right away. And she hung up.

I said to an empty line, Why can't anyone answer my fucking questions? Katya called to me from the other room, asking whom I was talking to.

I said, No one. That was the vet. The news on Winona is good.

That night I heated leftovers for dinner. Katya shared her chicken, and Lincoln his pizza, with the dog. She ate with gusto. She seemed better to me.

Sometimes one's imagination sees what it wants to see.

■ ■ ■

At eleven Lincoln walked into our room and said he couldn't sleep. I patted the bed next to me and he slid in. I got up and Googled Metacam. I spent the night collecting links to forward to our regular vet. By dawn I had become one of my clients, sending desperate letters full of legal theories cobbled together from stories told by inmates. I put on a suit and tie, flew to Dallas, and took a car to the courthouse.

Setting an execution date is about as momentous as clipping your toenails. The district attorney and I walked into Judge Tarsal's courtroom at nine. The judge was already sitting at the bench, chatting with a bailiff about where he was going fishing that weekend. Groups of defense lawyers were clustered off to the left, waiting to have the judge sign off on deals they had reached with prosecutors. The judge saw us walk in and asked us to approach. It was the middle of November. Under state law, execution dates must be set at least thirty days in advance. Kathy, the prosecutor, handed him an execution warrant, directing the warden to put Waterman to death on January 10, and asked him to sign. He asked me whether I had any objection. I said I did. I said, Your honor, I would like Mr. Waterman to be brought to the courtroom for this proceeding. If the district attorney is going to ask you to order that he be killed, and if you are going to do it, I think you should at least have to look him in the eyes. I think you should have to face the fact you are ordering the execution of a man who is in a very meaningful sense no longer the person he was when he participated in this horrible murder.

I like this judge. He is a good and decent man. I almost felt bad shoveling the entire responsibility onto him. He was only a foot soldier. He had no power, and I knew that, but my salve for impotence is to scream at whoever has to listen.

The judge turned to the district attorney. She was built like a low-slung ranch-style house from the 1950s. She had a flip hairstyle I had not seen since I watched Marlo Thomas on *That Girl* when I was in elementary school. She was wearing perfume that made her smell like my grandmother and caused my head to throb. She was wearing a brown suit with yellow vertical stripes that were failing their assignment if their job was to hide her girth. She reminded me of a shot putter gone soft. The seam running down the middle of the back of her jacket was stretched so tight I could see individual threads straining not to break. Maybe the stripes were canary. Her voice sounded like an ice pick in my brain. I would have felt that way even if I loved her, which would have been the opposite of how I actually felt.

The prosecutor insulted me once, two years before. My memory for slights is elephantine.

She said, Your honor, the professor's book says he believes in throwing sand in the gears of justice. This is all about throwing sand. It's delay for the sake of delay. Don't let him get away with it. The judge looked at me.

I said, Judge, in the first place, she's a poor reader, or maybe she didn't actually read the book. I didn't say I believe in throwing sand. But either way, I'm not here for a literary seminar. You are about to sign an order telling my client he will be dead in sixty days while the Supreme Court has not even ruled on his appeal. You are about to tell him this will be his last Christmas. I just think you should have to look at him and explain why it is acceptable to execute someone in America while his case is still pending.

He said, Your client would be shackled to the floor of an un-air-conditioned van for the five-hour drive from the prison to here. The transport team will probably stop at a McDonald's and have Quarter Pounders and fries in the air-conditioning while he swelters outside. I do not want to torture him just to tell him to his face that there is nothing I can do.

I didn't argue. The judge signed the order. The district attorney walked out without saying good-bye.

called my office at the university and asked my assistant to cancel my appointments. When I landed in Houston I drove straight to the prison. In Livingston, two miles down the road from death row, I stopped at Florida's for a late lunch. I don't eat lunch. I was there purely for the sake of delay.

The crowd was not exactly mixed. There was one black guy wearing a suit, two Hispanic guys wearing overalls, and fifteen or twenty mostly white corrections officers. I ordered a burger and onion rings. I took two bites and wrapped up the rest for dinner. I refilled my coffee for the third time. I noticed a corrections officer with captain's bars staring at me. When I caught his eye, he looked away. I left a 30 percent tip and walked outside. The smell of a wood fire reminded me of burning flesh, and I wondered what I would order for my last meal. I lifted the hatch of my car to make sure there was nothing there I didn't want the guards at the prison to see when they searched it. I turned and the captain from inside was standing by my side. He addressed me by name. He said, I hear Waterman's got a date.

Word travels fast.

He said, Yes sir, it does. The three others who'd been sitting at his table stepped outside. He said, Waterman's a good man. There's some of us who'd like to help. He looked back over his shoulder. He opened the door to a truck parked next to me and got in. The others joined him. They bounced out of the oyster-shell-covered parking lot and turned south toward the prison. I wrote down the truck's license plate number and followed them down the road.

In the visiting area Officer Scott asked me whom I wanted to see. When I plan to meet with more than one inmate, I prefer to get the more depressing visit out of the way first. Starret was crazy. Waterman would be dead in eight weeks. Hello, Sophie's choice. I said, How 'bout you choose for me today.

To prepare for my visit with Starret I read the transcript of the competency hearing. Cara had called the clerk at the court of appeals to ask for it. We assumed the court of appeals had the documents, because that court had upheld the lower court's decision allowing Starret to volunteer. How else could they agree Starret was competent without reviewing what he and the psychologist had said during the hearing? But the clerk at the court of appeals said they did not have the transcript. So we called the lower court, thinking it must have been returned. The clerk in the lower court told us they did not have it either. In fact, she said, a transcript had never been prepared. That seemed impossible. We tracked down the court reporter who had been present during the proceedings and asked him about it. He said, I never prepared a transcript. Nobody asked me to.

Every morning I wake up convinced nothing can surprise me, and every afternoon, something does. The court of appeals had ruled that Starret was competent to waive his appeals without even reviewing the facts of the case. We ordered a copy of the transcript ourselves. Cost is based on length. This one was going to be cheap. The hearing lasted less than an hour. Starret testified for thirty minutes, under questioning from the attorney general and the judge. I know his lawyer was in the room, because the documents say he was, but he did not ask a single question. Starret was asked how he spends his days, how much he sleeps, what he likes to eat, who comes to visit him, what magazines or books he reads, and whether he is sorry for what he did. He said he was. Then a psychologist testified for almost twenty minutes. The doctor had never actually met Starret. Instead, he reviewed a dozen documents and listened to Starret's testimony. He opined that Starret seemed perfectly competent to him. No one cross-examined him. No one asked him how many psychologists diagnose a man they have never met. The judge ruled Starret was competent to waive his appeals.

Before Starret picked up the phone he held his head in both his hands and scratched his scalp. He moved his lips like he was reciting a silent prayer. He was about my height but weighed probably fifty pounds less. His prison jumpsuit looked like it was hanging on broomsticks. We talked for nearly two hours. He described to me the days leading up to his crime. He had been on a weeklong meth binge. He claimed he had not slept in four days. His girlfriend lived with her mother. The mother did not like him. He broke into the house intending to confront her, but he fell asleep. He woke up because the cat jumped onto the bed. He heard the front door open and worried the cat would give away his presence. So he strangled the cat. He put the dead animal under the bed and hid in the shower. The person who had entered the house was his girlfriend's sister. He had sex with her. He said it was consensual. She was thirteen. The mother came home. Starret confronted her in the kitchen. He said she did not seem surprised to see him. Her calmness made him mad. A cat jumped up onto the table. He wondered how the cat had come back to life. It was staring at him and speaking a language he couldn't understand. He grabbed the cat around the throat and started to squeeze. His girlfriend's mother tried to stop him. He grabbed a knife from the counter. He stabbed her twenty-one times while her daughter fled through the bedroom window. When he was finished, he cut off her ponytail and put it in his pocket. Covered with blood, he walked to the corner and waited for the bus. He was the only passenger. The driver was watching him in the mirror. He got off at the next stop. He was arrested later that day.

I told Starret his sister had called and asked me whether I would represent her. She wanted to try to intervene in Starret's case and force him to pursue his appeal. He said, Ain't no need for that. I wrote the judge and told him I changed my mind. Miss Cara tole me you'd be my lawyer if I changed my mind. Is that right?

Death row inmates do not get to choose their lawyers. They get whomever the judge appoints. I told Starret I would ask the judge to appoint me, but I could not guarantee he would. Then I said, Your real problem, though, is that you've waived your appeal, and you won't get any lawyer at all unless a judge agrees to let you unwaive them. That means you will need a stay of execution, otherwise you'll be dead before anything can be filed. You follow me? He said he did but he looked like an art major listening to a lecture on differential equations. I said, I'll try to persuade a court to let you do that, but I'm not optimistic.

He said, You ain't what?

I said, I do not think there is a good chance you will get a stay of execution. I'll try my best, but we probably will fail. If we do manage to pull off a miracle, though, I can't make any promises about what will happen next.

He said, That's cool. I appreciate you trying to help. Waterman says you solid.

I said, He says what?

He said, You know, you'll do what you say, you feel me?

I nodded. I asked him whether there was anything else he needed. He said, You think you can get me something to sleep? I need to get me some sleep, man.

Death row has three levels. Level 1 is for the inmates who are well behaved. Level 3 is for the incorrigible. Level 2 is in between. Prisons are noisy places, but I had not heard of inmates on Level 1 being unable to sleep. I asked Starret whether they had moved him. He said, Nope. I'm in my same house.

So why can't you sleep?

'Cause they don't stop talking to me.

I said, Who doesn't?

Starret put down the phone and looked back over his shoulder. He craned forward and tried to look behind me. He leaned toward the glass and started to talk. I pointed to the phone he had put down and he picked it back up. He told me prison officials had put speakers inside the walls of his cell. He said, They use 'em to tell me shit. They're tryin' to help me out. I asked him who. He said it was guards, his daughter, even the warden. They offered him rewards if he would do certain things. He said the warden told him he would get moved to a cell with a view of a courtyard if he could sit motionless for an hour. So he sat still for ninety minutes. He said, But the motherfuckers didn't do like they promised. They're just fuckin' with me, man.

He told me he was through playing along. He just needed pills to help him sleep. He said, Man, I gotta sleep.

There are, of course, no cells on death row with courtyard views.

I had brought a copy of the transcript from the competency hearing. I opened to the page where the psychologist stated his name and held up the paper to the glass. I said, Have you ever met this guy? Starret looked at the page.

He said, I can't read that, man.

I said, You can't read?

He said, I can read. I just can't see that. It's all wiggly and shit, you feel me?

Starret had a pair of horn-rimmed glasses pushed up onto his head. I thought he might have forgotten they were there. I tapped my temple then motioned to his head. He squinted and looked confused. I told him his glasses were on his head. He said, Naw, man, I don't wear those. They make me look like a motherfuckin' serial killer. I ain't no serial killer.

I told him the psychologist's name. He said, I never met the man.

I told him I'd file something for him in the next day or two and stood up to leave. He said, You gonna go see Waterman now? I said nothing. He said, That nigger shouldn't even be in here. You tell him I'll catch up with his black ass later on. He touched his fist to the glass.

■ ■ ■

117

Before a seven-year drought parched western Colorado a decade ago, Katya and I took a weeklong trip on the Dolores, a 250-mile stretch of undammed river that runs north through the Dolores Canyon before turning west into Utah and flowing into the Colorado near the Dewey Bridge. We paddled the swollen river from morning until lunch, then hiked in the afternoons in canyons that still hide petroglyphs and twelfth-century Anasazi arrowheads.

It was six months before Peter learned he had cancer. I had never been in those canyons before, but I could tell from photos he would love them. We asked him to join us. He said no. He didn't want to spend a week on a raft, and he didn't want to run class IV rapids in a kayak. But he had another idea. He and Irmi used to take Katya and Phil skiing in Durango, less than an hour to the east. So before our river trip, Katya, Winona, and I spent two days hiking with Peter on the Colorado Trail.

I talked to him the night before Waterman got his date. He said, *I had a dream last night about our trip to Durango. Whenever I would stop to rest or drink, Winona would put her paw on my back. Do you remember that?*

I said, Are you talking about something from your dream?

He said, *No, it didn't happen in my dream. It happened on the trail. Do you*

118

remember Winona doing that? I thought it was odd. I forgot all about it until last night. I think she was trying to tell me something.

I said, I don't remember. What are you talking about?

He said, *Dogs can smell cancer.*

I said, I think they can smell lung cancer if they smell your breath and colorectal cancer if they smell your shit. I've never heard that they can smell melanoma.

He said, *Odor is odor. You and I have perhaps 5 million olfactory receptors in our noses. Winona has more than 200 million. Her actions weren't purposeless. She perceived something unusual. She was warning me of a danger even without knowing what it was, and I ignored her.*

I said, I don't think so. A couple of years ago I thought it would be neat to teach Winona to track. I bought a shelf of books and followed all the steps. She didn't really take to it very well.

He said, *No one is more dubious of exotic claims than I. Yet it's one thing to be skeptical. It's another to be so committed to skepticism that you close your eyes to contrary evidence.*

I've learned not to argue with people who say they see Jesus in a piece of burned toast. Either they're charlatans, and they know the truth already, or they're desperate, and they don't want to know. So I didn't tell him how, when I had tried to teach Winona to track, she couldn't even find a bacon-wrapped pork chop. After two weeks of futility, I gave away the books.

I said, Okay, I'll try to keep them open.

He said, *Give that dog a hard pet for me and tell her I'm sorry.*

Waterman came out. I told him the DA had given him a date. He shook his head and exhaled. He sagged just a little. He said, Guess you picked the wrong horse, huh?

From the day I had been appointed to represent Waterman, Jeffrey, Cara, and I, and the investigators working with us, had heard rumors there were at least half a dozen guards who would sign affidavits saying Waterman should not be executed. They would say he is not dangerous in prison and wouldn't be dangerous on the outside, either. Running into the captain at Florida's was providence telling me I needed to run those traps.

Of course, I don't believe in providence, but I had no other arrows left in the quiver. Besides, that angle looked more and more promising, and it was not just because it was the only angle left. We'd heard he would break up fights between inmates, counsel the young guys, white, black, or brown, and that on at least one occasion he had come to the rescue of a guard in trouble. A lieutenant had wanted Waterman to talk to young prisoners in general population, give them a sort of scared-straight pep talk. Waterman said he would do it, until the warden scuttled the idea. He was not bookish by any means, but he was getting his GED by mail, for no apparent reason, considering he'd be leaving prison in the back of a hearse.

Our facts looked good. All we needed was to find the people who could provide them and construct a legal theory where they mattered.

At one of our earliest strategy sessions, when Jeffrey and Cara first said they wanted us to prove that the jurors who believed Waterman would be dangerous were wrong, they proposed reinterviewing all the jurors to ask them whether, if they had known then what they know now, they would sentence Waterman to die. They wanted to pin our hopes—Waterman's hopes—on the fact he was the very opposite of dangerous, and that even the jurors who sent him to death row realized that now. I thought it was a losing argument.

I said to them, It's an interesting theory, but no. In the first place, I don't think the guards will come through. They're happy to talk as long as you're buying the beer and it doesn't cost them anything. Once they start worrying about their jobs, they lose their tongues. Plus, even if I'm wrong and they do sign affidavits, the legal argument is too complex. Occam's razor, folks. The simplest argument here is that the victim was already dead when Waterman shot her, and a competent lawyer would have proved that.

I've said before that a big difference between being a death penalty lawyer and being any other kind of lawyer is that other lawyers focus on where they are. If you are in the trial court, you focus on that. Court of appeals, focus on that. For a death penalty lawyer, you need to think far ahead, because it often doesn't matter if you win in the trial court. The appellate courts take away victories out of sheer hostility to your clients. Look ahead, look ahead. That's my mantra.

But in shaping our strategy for Waterman, I had forgotten my own advice. I got wedded to a theory that the trial judge bought—as he should have, considering we were right—but that the court of appeals would contort itself to reject. I should have known that would happen. How could I expect others to listen to me if I couldn't heed myself?

It can be difficult to acknowledge a mistake when your mistake is going to cost someone his life. But it was both too late and too early to flog myself for it now. I needed to focus on Plan B. I said to Waterman, I did pick the wrong horse, but the other one is still in the barn, saddled up and ready to ride. I need you to tell me the name of every guard you've known since you've been here who would say something good about you.

For two hours I coaxed names out of him. It was close to useless. *Sergeant Scott, Lieutenant Greevey, Officer Black.* Even knowing whether these guards were black or white, how was I going to find them with no first names, no addresses, and, in many cases, no current place of employment?

I said, Lucky we have a month.

He said, I ain't worried none. What happens happens. Buddhism is all about going wherever the river takes you.

I said, You're Buddhist now?

He said, No, not really. Don't mean I cain't learn something from 'em.

I smiled and stood up to leave. Waterman said, Please tell Jeffrey and Cara I said hello.

Walking back to my car I could hear dogs yelping, wishing some inmates would escape so they could get out of their pens and put their noses on the ground. I looked up at the watchtower and saw a guard leaning forward on the rail, a bolt-action rifle cradled across his forearms, staring at an empty yard. A guard buzzed me through the gate and handed me my driver's license. At my car, I found a piece of lined paper, torn from a spiral notebook, rolled and tucked inside the door handle. There was a seven-digit phone number, written in pencil. I assumed the area code was local. I looked to my left and right, then behind me. If there was anyone watching me, he was hiding. Or she. I folded the paper in half, then in half again, and put it in the back right pocket of my jeans.

On the drive back to Houston I called Waterman's daughter, Sharice. She was in college at Oklahoma State, majoring in social work. When I was first appointed Waterman's lawyer, I would call her mom twice a year or so with updates, and ask to talk to her. When Sharice was in high school, she let me. I'd been calling her a few times a year ever since. She seemed curious about her dad, asked to see photos of him and how he was doing. Once she asked for his address but if she ever wrote him, neither she nor Waterman told me about it.

I told her about Waterman's father, her granddad, and about Waterman's request that she write. I told her how he hoped to pass on some lesson from a father to a daughter before he was gone. She listened so wordlessly I was not sure she was there. I said, Did you hear me?

She said, Yes. I thought I could hear her sniffle, and she asked what would happen next. I told her I would ask the Supreme Court to review the case, but it probably wouldn't, and that he'd get executed right on schedule.

■ ■ ■

Death row is in a dry Texas county. The guards who watch over murderers all day have to drive thirty miles at night to get a beer.

I crossed the county line, and there was the liquor store, like Sabbath manna. I pulled into the dirt parking lot littered with cigarette butts, crushed beer cans, and empty half-pint bottles of gut-rot rye. Sharice was quiet. She whispered, It's almost Christmas. An eighteen-wheeler carrying timber blew up a cloud of red dust like a western.

Sharice asked whether there was any chance the parole board would recommend that his death sentence be replaced with a life sentence. I wondered how she knew about the parole board. I said, No. I don't think so.

I could hear her start to cry.

I said, But you never know.

Back at the office, Jeffrey, Cara, and I sat down with Juanita, an investigator I pulled off everything else she was working on, and two second-year law students. I figured we had twenty interviews to conduct: twelve jurors and six or eight guards. We also had to write up the argument. I said, Jeffrey can help me write. Y'all hit the road. Prison guards and jurors will talk more to women. Wear suits for the jurors, not for the guards. We'll meet every morning at eight to map out the day.

Cara said, What about Starret?

Fuck, I forgot all about him.

Cara said, We figured. Jeffrey and I drafted something. I'll send it to you.

■ ■ ■

When I got home from the office Katya was in front of the computer reading about interleukin-2, an experimental treatment that might help the body's own immune system attack melanoma. She had a legal pad on her lap. I kissed her and picked it up. She'd written *ipilimumab*. I said, What's that? She told me it's a drug that targets CTLA-4, a protein that suppresses the T-cell immune response. Having suppressed T-cells might help melanoma cells survive; ipilimumab might mean more activated T-cells; more activated T-cells might mean less melanoma; hence, ipilmumab might be good. I said, Do they use this at Anderson?

She didn't take her eyes off the screen. She said, I feel completely alone. When I talk to him, he does not think about what I am saying. He thinks about how to respond.

I wrapped my arms around her, and we sat in silence. One thing I've learned is that in the face of tragedy you are powerless to prevent, there's no greater empathy than quiet.

My stomach growled. I said, Apparently I'm starving.

She said, Me too.

We drove to Goode Company seafood and sat at the bar. She was eating oysters. I was eating ceviche. We were splitting a plate of fried tomatoes. But neither of us was saying a word. I knew what she was thinking about. She knew what I was thinking about, too. I was wondering how long I would have to talk to Starret in a public setting before his tenuous grasp on reality became apparent. I didn't think a judge would give me longer than about ten minutes, which was probably a couple of hundred minutes fewer than what I needed. She was thinking about losing her dad before she was ready for him to be gone. Finally Katya said, If you can get through to your crazy client, maybe you can work on Papa for me. She smiled, but it wasn't happiness.

There was a difference, though, between her dad and Starret. Starret was nuts. Her dad was just angry. My clients count down the days to their deaths. Peter counted them down in reverse. He had said to me, *I kept my end of the bargain. The cosmos reneged.* I had told him the fact he was angry didn't make folding up his tent noble. He said, *I am not swallowing a bottle of pills or jumping off a roof. I am not calling Dr. Kevorkian. I've simply decided to spend my days living. It escapes me how that is tantamount to folding up a tent.* He was seething. I swear I could feel heat coming off his neck. I told him I wasn't convinced. Maybe he was doing it to live more fully. Maybe he was doing it to quit living sooner. I had said to him, Angry men are unhappy even on mountaintops. He said, *Yes. That is true.*

I said to Katya, Your dad is more stubborn than Starret, but he loves you and Phil and your mom more than he hates his life. Based on my track record, I think you might have a better chance of getting through to him than I will. She smiled again. This time it was happiness, or something close.

■ ■ ■

hitewater kayakers measure river volume in CFS, how many cubic feet of water flow past a given point every second. Optimal recreational flow on the lower Guadalupe in central Texas is four or five hundred CFS. But the remnants of a late-season storm had parked over Austin for three straight days, and the Guad was running at over 100,000 CFS. My friend Craig called me and said, DPS has blocked the access road, but I know how we can get to the put-in.

At that level there is no definable river, only a vast wall of water rushing downstream. Piles of uprooted trees and severed limbs create porous dams kayakers call strainers. The only skill required in such conditions is avoiding those strainers, because if you get swept into one, you will drown.

I called Peter and told him he would not get another chance like this even if he lived to be a hundred. He said, *I do not think this is wise, but if we can pick up barbeque in Luling on the way, I am open to persuasion.*

Which is how he, Katya, and I came to be eating brisket and ribs in the car on the way to meeting Craig at a place in Gruene where there used to be a bridge. We hiked upriver through the brush, got in our boats, and seal launched into the current. Peter immediately flipped. I saw him come out of his boat and saw Katya race to catch up with him. She reached him in the middle of the river and angled her boat so she could tow him to shore, but when he grabbed the loop on her stern, she flipped too.

Now they were both swimming in the middle of the roiling river, and even Michael Phelps could not have competed with that current. Katya had one hand locked on her father's life vest but was struggling to swim them both to shore. Craig and I caught up to them at the same time. They took ahold of the grab loops on our boats and we paddled them to the bank. When Peter finally caught his breath he said, *I knew this was a bad idea. I am getting out. That is plenty enough for me.*

Katya said, I'm going to stay here with Papa. If you two are crazy enough to get back in, and lucky enough not to kill yourselves, come pick us up when you're done. As Craig and I were sealing ourselves back into our boats, she said, You're really going? I kissed her and told her we'd be fine.

It didn't take us long to run the river. We saw three boaters surfing on a massive wave right below a rapid called Slant that didn't used to be there, and sheriffs' deputies occasionally hollered at us from the bank that the river was closed. We saw two washing machines, three cars, and one small cabin, all washing downstream toward Seguin. A trip that normally takes close to three hours took us twenty-one minutes. Sitting on the bank at the takeout Craig said, Dude, that was pretty stupid.

We got in my truck and headed up to where we'd left my wife. It was raining lightly. At a stoplight in the town square, an old man in a wheelchair was rolling himself across the intersection. One of the small front wheels fell into a pothole, and he was stuck. Cars steered around him. When the light changed to red and then back to green, the backed-up traffic didn't move. Nobody honked, either. Everyone just stood there. Craig and I hopped out. The man had three or four days of gray beard growth, and a plastic grocery bag filled with cans balanced on his lap. He said, Seem to have got myself into a pickle. His eyes sparkled. Craig and I pushed him onto the sidewalk. He said, Thanks young fellas, and he rolled on down the street.

The entire episode took maybe five minutes, but what happened in those five minutes couldn't have mattered more. That night Katya told me what she and her dad had talked about. She reminded him how he had saved her from drowning when she had been trapped in a recirculating hole below a flat head dam on this very river. She told him that everything she had learned about trying to be a good person she had learned from him. But she and her brother, she said, had so much more to learn. She told him about the places she wanted them to see, the things she hoped they would discuss.

She told me he parried and resisted every word, up until the moment Craig and I arrived. She had just told him he and her mom were like a single organism that would die if he gave up. She told me he said his wife's name, *Irmi*, then said, *Enough, liebe. I will agree to one more round.*

Katya said he was crying when he said it, his voice a whisper. She said, I could barely hear him over your broken muffler. You really should get that fixed.

I told her about our trip down the river and our encounter with the man in the wheelchair. She said, So I had enough time to get through to Papa because of the extra few minutes that man bought me.

I said, So it appears. Quite a coincidence, huh?

＊ ＊ ＊

have a former student named Li. In law school, he worked with me on capital cases. After graduation, he gave it up for money. Now he's a successful patent lawyer. When he comes to town we like to play chess and trade war stories. He called on a perfect winter day, cloudless and crisp, and asked if I had time to meet him at McElroy's. McElroy's has Blue Moon on tap. I told him I'd be there in twenty minutes.

In law school, he had worked on cases of several mentally ill inmates. I told him about Starret. He said, In China, the system for protecting intellectual property is medieval compared to the United States, but the death penalty regime seems not so different.

I said, It's possible you've spent too much time listening to me rail.

He was playing black but crushing me anyway. I was looking at the board, seeing if there was any way for me to salvage a draw. We had just ordered our second beers when my phone rang. It was Jeffrey.

He said, Darnell Springsteen's mom just called up here looking for you. You want me to give her your cell?

I said, God no. I'll be back on campus in ten minutes.

Three months earlier, after the Supreme Court decided not to hear his appeal, Springsteen's lawyer called to ask whether we had any good ideas for what he could do next. Cara, Jeffrey, and I discussed it and came up with no good idea. I told him we couldn't think of anything to do. Then Springsteen himself wrote, begging us to help him. His handwriting slanted across the page at thirty degrees. The letter was a single unindented, unpunctuated paragraph. It made no sense at all, but there was no mistaking his intent. At the end he had written HELP ME in all upper case.

Although other states have the death penalty, no place carries it out like Texas. Experienced death penalty lawyers who come to Texas know the law, but not the psychology. Jeffrey moved here from Florida. A few months after he started working for me, his first client got executed. He came to work the next morning with red swollen eyes and asked me how people keep doing this work, execution after execution. I said, Work on developing a cold cold heart, pal.

He said, Your advice is a Hank Williams song?

I said, You're going to fit right in here. And he did. The day after his next client got put to death, he was the first person to the office. I found him writing an appeal for an inmate scheduled for execution in a month.

I wrote back to Springsteen and said there was nothing we could do.

Springsteen and a career criminal named Samantha had kidnapped an elderly woman, apparently intending to ransom her. It was all Samantha's idea. Springsteen himself couldn't define ransom if you gave him a multiple-choice test with only a single option. They grabbed the woman from her stoop, taped her mouth shut, and stuffed her in the trunk of Samantha's car. They drove to a motel. Springsteen asked Samantha who they were going to call and ask for money. Samantha said, We gonna akse her exactly that question.

They opened the trunk and the woman was dead. Samantha

decided they would still make the ransom demand by calling the woman's home number and talking to whoever answered, but they might as well dispose of the body, so they drove to a bridge over the Trinity River, tied the body to a cinder block, and heaved the woman into the water.

Except it turned out she wasn't dead. She'd had a heart attack, but was still breathing. Her body surfaced the next day. The medical examiner said she had drowned. Springsteen actually had some compelling legal issues, including that he was almost certainly retarded. But he had taken an elderly woman from her rocking chair and thrown her still alive into a river with a brick tied around her waist. Do you care he was retarded, that he did what he did because Samantha told him to? If you answered no you have company. The judges didn't either.

I resigned the game I was going to lose anyway and told Li I had to run. He said, Are you working on the case?

I said, Not exactly.

When I walked into my office, Springsteen's mother was on hold, waiting for me. She and her daughter Lisa, Springsteen's older sister, were staying at a cheap motel in Livingston, Texas, home of death row. They had spent four hours that day with Springsteen at the prison, talking to him on a phone through a thick Plexiglas bulletproof window in a Lysol-smelling room with cracked linoleum floors and walls painted the color of key lime pie. They would spend two more hours with him the next day. His mom would tell her son good-bye, but she wouldn't get to kiss him or hold his hand. Prison officials would load Springsteen into a windowless van for the ninety-minute drive to the Walls Unit, where they would stick him in a holding cell eight steps from the execution chamber, feed him a final meal, strap him to the gurney, and put him to death.

Desperation and I are on intimate terms, but hysterical people usually don't make sense, and Springsteen's mother was well past the margin of rationality. I asked her three times to repeat what she was saying. She was sputtering and sobbing and I couldn't understand a word. I was getting frustrated. I wanted to be sitting outside drinking my beer and smoking my cigar. I listened hard but still couldn't understand, so I just said, Ms. Springsteen, I am sorry that there is nothing we can do for your son. His appeals are over. Unfortunately, it is too late to file anything else.

I heard the phone clatter to the ground. I heard her saying, No no no over and over again. I heard her say, You said he would help us. I heard her daughter saying, Calm down, Mama, calm down. It will be okay. Then Lisa picked up the phone. She said, Sir, how can they take him tomorrow when the court just turned down his appeal today?

What was she talking about? I had the history of his case on my computer screen. I told her the court of appeals had ruled against him thirteen months earlier and the Supreme Court had rejected his appeal a year after that. She said, But I sent them a new one.

I said, You did? Are you a lawyer?

No, sir.

I said, Well, the problem is that once the first appeal is decided, you can't file anything else without getting special permission.

She said, From who? Nobody tole me that. And his lawyer didn't do what Darnell asked him to.

I found myself thinking, Maybe I should ask the governor for a thirty-day reprieve. Maybe there is an issue hidden here somewhere we can try to use to get a stay. I said, I know how terrible that is, but the rules require that you file your appeal in advance. It is just too late now to do anything.

She said, That ain't right. It ain't. I heard her mother talking between sobs. Lisa took the phone away from her mouth and said something back. I wanted to hang up. I looked out my window and could see the Campari umbrella Li and I had been sitting beneath ten minutes before. Lisa got back on the phone and said, Cain't I file my own appeal?

I have four younger brothers. We recently wrote a trivia book with questions like: Name the only two people ever to baby-sit for us more than once. (Answer: my mom's brother and sister.) When I was twelve, Linda from down the street baby-sat one Saturday night. As soon as my parents left for dinner, we five boys went into their bedroom and locked the door. We played a game called King of the Mountain. This involved jumping on the bed and pushing each other off, until only one person remained. Linda banged on the door. I told my brothers to ignore her. Somebody pushed someone into a painting, and the glass in the frame shattered. The bedroom door swung open. Linda had called her mother, who knew how to jimmy open locks. While Linda's mother was telling me my plan was a terrible idea, that I should instead confess my error and say I was sorry, I used Saran Wrap to re-create the glass.

When my parents got home an hour later, we were pretending to be asleep. It was the earliest we had gone to bed on a Saturday night in years. I heard my dad say to my mom, Honey, come in here and look at this. A moment later I felt him sitting on the edge of my bed. I kept my eyes pressed closed. He said, I expect more from you. Then he walked out of my room and gently closed the door. It made a soft *click* I can still hear, forty years later, every time I make a critical decision.

Springsteen grew up in Ouchita Parish, in northeast Louisiana. I heard Cajun in his sister's voice. I felt myself waver, like when you're walking across a balance beam, and you feel yourself start to fall before you actually do, when there is still time to save it, so you wave your arms and tighten your gut, but you overcorrect, and then there is no way to make it, and so you just give it up and drop.

But I did catch myself. Springsteen was a dead man. There was not a single thing we could do. We had Waterman's and Starret's fates in our hands, and there wasn't room on the raft for another. I didn't know Springsteen's mother or sister. I did not owe them anything. You can't tell others to nourish a cold cold heart if your own always melts from human breath.

I asked Lisa whether she had a computer. She said, Un-uh, but I got me some paper. Fifteen years ago, before courts accepted filings by email, we would transmit our eleventh-hour appeals by fax. She said, The motel says we can use their fax machine. But I don't know the number.

I found the fax number we used to use and gave it to her. I said, Ms. Springsteen, I am going to give you the number. But I don't want you to think this is going to work. I think you should tell your mother that she needs to tell Darnell good-bye, and that's what I think you should do, too. Nobody is at the Supreme Court right now to read what you send, and when they get there tomorrow, it won't make any difference. I'm going to give you the number, but I'm telling you it won't help.

She said, But it cain't hurt, right?

When I hung up the phone the moon had risen and Jeffrey and

Cara had gone. I picked up sushi on the way home and gave Lincoln a five-foot-tall stuffed version of Doc from the Seven Dwarfs, a gift from Li. Later, while Lincoln brushed his teeth, I read an interview with the comedienne Margaret Cho. Someone asked her what she would eat for her final meal. She said macaroni and cheese and fried chicken. She said, If I get executed, I figure it will be somewhere in the South, and I want to have the regional specialty. When I laughed out loud, Lincoln asked me what was so funny.

Nothing.

Dada, I think you are trying to protect me from something.

I said, Linco, I don't think you would think it's funny.

I don't know what it is, but you're protecting me. You don't always have to protect me, Dada.

The next morning when I got to my office I found a copy of Darnell Springsteen's sister's last frantic effort to save her brother's life. My assistant had left it in my chair. It was handwritten on an unlined page, full of exclamation points and underlined words. I wondered what the clerk at the Supreme Court thought when he saw it. I wondered if it made him cry. It was not an appeal. It was a primal wail of pain. I'm sure no justice ever read it.

■ ▦ ▨

I submitted to the chemo because Katya persuaded me the part of my life I own is exceeded by the sum of what others own, and that by surrendering so soon I was inflicting on Irmi an injury I had the power to avoid. When I agreed, I understood intellectually what would happen, but I did not truly understand. Chemotherapy is poison. The doctors who administer it are like gardeners. Through a process of trial and error they try to mix a perfect poison, one that will kill the weeds but not the shrubs. But to the poison, a plant is a plant, a cell is a cell. So the gardeners and the doctors tinker. They make fine adjustments to kill some things and not others. It is neither art nor science, just crude, continual recalibration.

I feel a hole where my liver used to be. I feel it growing back. I also feel cancer, like a grain of sand in your eye, coursing through my veins.

My brain feels shrunken. I cannot form thoughts. I cannot listen to Bach. I read a sentence and when I look up I cannot remember it. When I wake up in the morning and push the sheet aside, I do not recognize my own legs. I do not even try to imagine running a mile again one day. I try to imagine walking half a block.

Irmi's food, which used to give me such pleasure, tastes like metal shavings. An open bottle of champagne on the counter across the room makes me retch. I sit on my stool in the shower and scrub myself raw, yet still I feel filthy, like I am rinsing the wrong side of a window. I brush my teeth until my gums bleed and my saliva tastes like sour milk.

I am nearing the end of the chaos, meaning I am nearing the end. I can feel that. On my fifth day home I could not sit inside any longer. I had to be on the water. All I planned to do was float, but the winds were strong. I thought I could surf. Irmi was inside doing laundry. I climbed on to the board and headed toward the cove, and I fell almost immediately. I couldn't pull the sail back out of the water, so I just lay down on my belly and paddled back to the dock. I looped a line around a cleat because I was too tired to haul the board out of the water, and when I looked up, Irmi was standing there. Her cheeks were crimson. Her lips quivered. She repeated my name three times and I could not meet her eyes. By the time I got up the ladder, she was inside. There was a towel on the floor next to the door.

When I walked in she did not speak. She was sitting in the living room reading, or pretending to, her back to me. She had poured herself a glass of wine. It was not yet nine in the morning.

I once heard a therapist say that anger is never the first emotional reaction one has to a circumstance. Something else comes first, maybe jealousy, perhaps envy. Only then comes the anger. I recognize this as my final November. Thanksgiving will be my last. My final Christmas I may have already had.

The tumors are in my brain. I knew this before the scan results arrived last night. The film reveals three. How many more are too small to see is anybody's guess.

Yes I am angry, but not because life is unfair. I am angry because there is no progress, because nothing has worked, because I actually feel the end, although I cannot explain it. I am angry because I am frightened. Wouldn't you be?

■ ■ ■

On Thanksgiving I sat next to my bubbe. She was getting old by then, eighty-three if my memory serves. She said, Yesterday I was at the Jumbo supermarket and bought ten pounds of sweet potatoes.

My aunt walked over to say hello. She asked why I didn't have any sweet potatoes on my plate. I told her I do not care for them. When she walked away, my bubbe whispered, I don't like them either.

I said, But you just told me you bought ten pounds yesterday.

She said, They were only nineteen cents a pound.

When I told the story to Peter the following day, he didn't even smile.

It was the Friday after Thanksgiving, and we were at the lake. Irmi had prepared all the traditional favorites for a day-late holiday. Usually before a meal Peter would lead us on what he called a short walk. It might last for two hours. This day he said, *I'm not feeling well. Can we skip the walk?* And he sat down in the rocking chair without waiting for an answer.

The first sign of brain tumors had been sudden seizures. After the first fall, he put a stool in the shower. The oncologist prescribed a medicine to prevent them. The seizures stopped, but he developed vertigo so severe he could not stand. That morning Irmi found him doubled over with stomach pain, unable even to sit up, less than an hour after he took his morning dose. She paged the doctor three times in an hour. He finally called her back. He had prescribed a dose of the antiseizure medication based on a man of Peter's height and weight. But that calculation assumes normal liver function. Three-fourths of Peter's liver was gone. The overdose of the medicine was making Peter's world spin faster than it had before. The doctor instructed Irmi to break the pills in thirds.

I said, Seriously? In thirds? She thanked him for returning the call. He did not say you're welcome, and he didn't say he was sorry.

Peter said, *I do not know whether it was the Babylonians or the Indians who invented the concept of zero, but I believe it was the Chinese who conjured up negative numbers. And now I have proof they are real. My doctors are making me worse. They have pushed me lower than zero.* He thanked us for coming, then he excused himself from the table and went off to bed.

■ ■ ■

tarret was going to be the last execution victim of the year. We had filed a motion for rehearing the court of appeals, asking them to reconsider their determination that Starret was competent to surrender his appeals. There are seventeen judges on the court of appeals, but they usually sit in panels of three to hear cases. We had filed our motion with the entire court. I wanted all the judges to know that three of their colleagues had upheld a decision allowing a mentally ill inmate to waive his appeal without even bothering to read the transcript of the proceeding.

As it turned out, they didn't care. As far as the judges on the court of appeals were concerned, they did not need to read the transcript of the competency hearing. They did not need to read it because it did not matter whether Starret was competent. It didn't matter whether he was competent because they had no intention of letting him turn back on his appeals, which he would undoubtedly lose anyway, because what he had done was rape a thirteen-year-old girl and stab the girl's mother twenty-one times. Imagine that happening to your sister and your mom and see how sympathetic you'd be to the recondite legal claims articulated by the lawyer representing the thug.

Of course, you're not a judge.

Katya and I were reading a story in the *New York Times Magazine* about the two men who broke into a home in Cheshire, Connecticut. They beat the homeowner, a doctor, leaving him for dead. They raped and murdered his wife. They raped and murdered his two daughters, stabbing them and setting them on fire.

Somehow the man survived. He crawled onto his driveway where a neighbor found him. The article was about how his life had still essentially ended. His loved ones were murdered. Years later he could still hear their screams.

I said to Katya, If this happened to you and Lincoln I'd smuggle a gun into the courtroom and kill the two men myself.

I have actually thought about this in great detail, considered how I would get the gun inside. I won't tell you how I could do it, but I could. I have no doubt. Katya said, I know.

But I am not a judge, either. I did not take an oath to set aside my passions and uphold the rule of law. I'm allowed to permit emotion to rout reason.

The clerk of the court called to say our motion had been denied. Cara, Jeffrey, and I sat down to discuss Plan B.

There wasn't a lot to discuss. We did not yet even have the file from the case. Starret's lawyer was supposed to deliver it later that day. Our knowledge of the facts was minimal to nonexistent. We did know two critical details: that a trial court had permitted a crazy man to waive his appeals, and that an appellate court had upheld that decision without even reviewing the case.

But, at least in my experience, moral outrage does not save lives. We needed a legal argument. I said, When the files get here, comb through them looking for every document that has anything at all to do with mental health. If we can convince the Supreme Court he really is unbalanced, maybe we'll get a stay.

At six Thursday evening, Starret's previous lawyer arrived at our office in a pickup truck with thirteen banker's boxes of documents loaded in the bed. Maybe he understood his filing system, but to us it was a mess. Materials from the state habeas appeal were next to reports from the pretrial investigation. Elementary school records were next to a biography of the federal judge printed off Wikipedia. The organization was neither chronological, nor substantive, nor alphabetical. If there was any logic to how the materials were arranged, it was a code I couldn't break. I asked Cara to have two students work nonstop organizing and indexing the thousands of pages. I said, I'd like it done no later than first thing Monday, but if it is ready sooner, call me immediately no matter what time it is.

■　■　■

Katya was lying on the sofa in the library when I got home. I could hear her talking on the phone. She hung up as I walked in and immediately started to cry. I said, What?

She said, I just spent twenty minutes on the phone with Papa. I called to tell him we were looking forward to being at the lake tomorrow. He said, *I was going to wait until then to tell you, Katya, but I am not having any more surgery.* I asked whether it was the doctor's recommendation or his self-managed treatment. He said, *This futile resistance is shortening my number of pleasant days, not giving me more.* I said, Isn't being alive pleasant? He said, *I blame only myself for succumbing to your browbeating. I should have trusted my judgment and savored my final days. Instead I have become an unhappy and desiccated man.*

I said to Katya, He actually used the word *browbeating?*

She said, Yes. I asked him how he thinks it makes Mama and Phil and me feel that your clients want to be with their families more than he wants to be with us. He said, *Maybe you should try listening harder to what I am telling you.* He had to be able to tell I was crying. Then he said good night and hung up the phone.

Katya said, Let's not go tomorrow.

I said, Let's go have dinner and talk about it.

We went to Brenner's and sat outside. Buffalo Bayou was swollen from two days of rain and running fast. A lone peacock strutted across the grassy hill and disappeared into a stand of cypress trees. There was an open fire pit burning a mix of hickory and pecan. We were drinking champagne and eating steak. Mine was cooked, hers was blue. I said, Moo, and speared an onion ring off her plate. I said, You want this, and she shook her head. My every effort at mirth was failing. I said, He is trying to push you away because he thinks that is better for you.

She said, So what am I supposed to do?

I said, Don't let him. Every time he pushes, hold on tighter.

Katya said, His anger is defeating my love. How is that possible?

I said, Waterman's daughter doesn't talk to him and that makes him depressed. Your dad is depressed so he doesn't want to talk to you. I think depression is the strongest force in the universe. It can destroy love and even human will. Say what you want to say, even if he tries not to hear it.

She said, It won't matter.

I said, It won't hurt.

She pushed her plate away. I held her right hand with my left and drank a snifter of cognac while I traced a circle in her palm with my thumb. When we got home she trudged upstairs, weary as a refugee. Before we went to sleep I kissed her deeply and held her face in my hands. I said, Everything will be okay.

It was a time in my life when I still confused comforting my wife with filling the silence. She was crying softly when I fell asleep.

T wo other couples were at the lake house when we got there the next day. Irmi had called in reinforcements to help get through to Peter. All three men were chemists for Shell, all three German. They had known each other forty years. Their wives were German, too. They were debating whether Germany should send troops to Iraq. Katya joined the argument. I just listened. I can't speak German.

My phone rang. Cara said, You won't believe this, but in the files we found a picture of the jury. One of the jurors must have had a Polaroid.

I said, Yeah?

She said, Twelve white faces.

Cara had called me on a Saturday afternoon because this was stunning and important. In the mid-1980s, the U.S. Supreme Court decided a case called *Batson v. Kentucky*. The Court ruled that prosecutors are not permitted to remove blacks from the jury on account of their race. They still do it routinely, of course, but they aren't supposed to, and if you can prove a *Batson* violation, your client gets a new trial.

Starret was tried in East Texas, in a county that is 60 percent black. The odds of having an all-white jury by sheer chance were like winning the Lotto twice. The inverse of that calculation meant that the odds of prosecutorial misconduct were substantial. But proving a so-called *Batson* violation is difficult and time-consuming. We would need to learn the race of the potential jurors the prosecutors struck, and we would need to try to figure out why they struck them. We would need to compare how the prosecutors questioned potential white jurors with how they questioned potential black jurors. And before we could do that, we would need to figure out the color of all the people questioned who were not on the jury. Putting together a *Batson* claim takes months. We had less than three days.

I said, Have the students do the research on who is what color. Write a claim with whatever you can learn. Get it to me by noon Monday. We have to file by six.

She said, You think there's enough time?

I said, Nope. Tell whoever's working on it that the goal is neither completeness nor perfection. We don't need an A plus. We need a D minus. If Starret's still alive in a week, we'll make the claim better.

Even though Starret was not scheduled to die until Wednesday, I wanted to file the papers by Monday because the Texas court had a rule requiring that challenges to executions be filed forty-eight hours in advance. Lawyers who violate the rule are subject to a laundry list of sanctions, including jail and disbarment. The chief judge on the court had already publicly accused me of telling lies about her in an effort to get her removed from the bench. I didn't want to press the court's buttons. Cara said, We're on it.

The other two couples left. Peter asked whether I wanted to take a stroll while the coals burned down. I didn't. I said, Sure.

He said, *Will you smoke this cigar while we walk?* He handed me a Bolivar Robusto, a strong Cuban cigar that's one of my favorites. Peter used to tell me not to smoke.

I said, You want me to smoke this?

He said, *Now that my fate is sealed, I'm sampling sin. The secondhand smoke will please me.* I turned around and looked at Katya. She shrugged her shoulders and rolled her eyes. We crossed the street, walked across a meadow, and into the forest. We walked for twenty minutes. The only sounds were leaves crunching and Peter's heavy breathing. Then he said, *Last night I finished the book of Montaigne essays. In one Montaigne says that all human beings are double, so that we do not believe what we believe. It made me think of you, how I never know what you believe, how you disagree and argue just to test some hypothesis. Do you remember how that day on the salt flats you told me my commitment to environmentalism was a mere aesthetic choice, devoid of any moral value?*

I did remember. I nodded. He said, *That angered me, until I realized you were just pressing me to make the moral argument more perspicuous. It comforted me to know that you and I do not disagree on much that is fundamental. And that is why I am so troubled that we do not agree on who owns my life. Aren't all of us entitled to control our own destinies?*

He was breathing harder. I wasn't sure whether it was exertion or exasperation. He said, *I believe we are, but what is more, I do not think any other view is reasonable or legitimate. I do not see how you, a smart man, could hold it.* I started to say something until I remembered how my lame attempt to fill the silence the night before had resulted in an idiotic platitude. I wasn't angry. I just didn't have anything useful to say. I turned my head to the left and blew out a mouthful of smoke. Peter said, *I am the only person alive who experiences what I experience. The only one. Neither you nor Katya nor even Irmi can feel what is happening to me.* His voice was vibrating. What I had thought might be exasperation now seemed definitely closer to anger. *You all want me to stay alive, but that is because you want me to be in your lives. Of course that flatters me, and makes me happy and sad, but that desire does not give you a ballot, and even if it did, it is wrong to cast a vote that treats me as a means to your ends. I want to die with dignity, and you all are determined to thwart me.*

I tell Lincoln it's okay to make a mistake. It's not okay to make it twice. I still said nothing. Peter said, *Well?*

Perhaps my greatest weakness is taking the bait. I said, I know a woman who could not get pregnant. She and her husband traveled to fertility clinics for treatments in five different states. After three years and more than half a million dollars, success. In fact, too much success. Her obstetrician told her there were five fetuses developing. She and her husband decided to abort two of them. After all that time and money, they were spending more money to get rid of two babies. I'm not being critical here, just noting the irony.

In the moment I took to inhale, Peter said, *Does that have anything to do with what I said?*

I said, Not yet. Three healthy babies were born, two boys and a girl. They are in fourth grade. A month ago, the mother announced to the family that she is a lesbian. She packed her bags, kissed her kids, and moved into an apartment. Now, at six o'clock, instead of cooking dinner for her triplets, she's at happy hour at some gay bar looking to hook up.

I paused. Peter said nothing. I said, If living as a heterosexual woman was a lie to her, I think she should have kept living a lie a little longer, maybe not for the rest of her life, but for long enough for her kids to get through high school. I know the kids. They'll probably be fine eventually, but they are going to be good and fucked up for a while, and it could be a long while. I don't think she had the right to do that to them. You have responsibilities to other people. Some you choose, some you don't.

I looked at Peter. He did not look at me. His jaw muscle pulsed like he was chewing stale gum. I said, I think her choice was decadent. I think yours is too.

We were still walking. He kept looking straight ahead. He said, *Wow.* And then he said it again.

One thing I've learned is that there is a time to be silent and there's a time to hold nothing back. What I might not have learned is which is when.

We got back to the house and Peter told me he could grill the flank steak by himself. In the kitchen Irmi was cooking potatoes and Katya was dressing a salad. I poured a tall glass of Knob Creek. Katya looked at the amount of bourbon and said, Tough walk? I told her I'd tell her about it later.

Peter brought the meat in on a platter and sliced it thinly against the grain. He set it down on the counter, next to the other food, and over it squeezed a lime. He poured a tall glass of water, drank it all, and filled it again. He said, *I'm not feeling well. Please eat without me.* He carried his water into the bedroom and closed the door.

Katya and Irmi looked at me like I had answers, or possibly like I was to blame. I said, I might have gone a little too far, and I told them what had happened.

Irmi said nothing. She got up and walked to the bedroom. We could hear them talking, but not what they were saying. Katya picked up a slice of meat, took a bite, and pushed her plate away. She put her arm around my neck and pulled my head down to hers. She kissed my ear and said, Thank you.

■ ■ ■

hy can't you understand that when someone is having his last Thanksgiving or his final Christmas or his ultimate anything, he cannot help but focus on the fact it will be his last? I'm not mad anymore, not at you, just perplexed.

Last night, after I finally emerged from my snit, I finished The Crossing. *I dog-eared the page where McCarthy wonders whether people would choose to live their lives if they knew its details in advance. I made a list with five headings. I moved to a strange country, found my perfect soul mate, had two wonderful children, earned enough money to support my family, and planned how I would live the two decades after my retirement. I made some notes under each heading, except for the last. The border that separated my plans from my reality was a trip to a country doctor in a cookie-cutter strip center who cut out a lump I'd lived with for months and sent me to a specialist I didn't know who told me I would be dead in a year. I think McCarthy thinks most people would not want their lives. But I would. That's exactly why I'm angry.*

You can be a judgmental and pedantic son of a bitch. But I've come to think you might be at least a little bit right. The brain surgery has been rescheduled for Thursday.

This surgery I am doing for myself. I wish I could have it now. Apparently, however, I am not the only dying man my surgeon must attend to, so I must wait three more days. How significantly did the chemotherapy weaken my blood–brain barrier? How many more metastases will take root in the next seventy-two hours while I sit here, doing nothing, sliding passively toward death?

Why can no one tell me?

For the first time in my life I spend hours on end doing nothing, too tired to think, too bitter to love, too angry to speak. I'd prefer any death to this one. To die with a desiccated brain is the only death I fear. I've said it before but I feel the need to say it again because no truth seems greater to me: I must have done something truly evil to deserve this. When will I learn what it was?

▦　▦　▦

onday morning I taught my class at the law school, told my assistant I would be unreachable most of the afternoon, and went to the prison to see Starret. A potential *Batson* claim meant the last-minute litigation in his case could unfold differently from how I had previously described it to him. I wanted to make sure he understood what would be happening and was comfortable with it. He knew we were trying to allow him to retract his decision to waive his appeals, but he did not know—because we did not know—we might identify a promising legal claim.

Many death row inmates think they can manage their lawyers. They want to be consulted about their cases, like they're capable of offering meaningful advice. They believe they are part client and part colleague. They think their lawyers aren't doing their jobs, or that they have abandoned them, if the lawyers don't come to the prison every few weeks to visit.

I understand their frustration. If your life is in somebody else's hands, you'd like to know what those hands are doing all the time. But death row inmates are not lawyers, and their instructions to their attorneys about which claims to pursue is like a patient telling a doctor which medicine to prescribe. I go to the prison five or six times a year so my clients do not feel alone, so they know the lawyers in my office are working sixteen hours a day to save their lives, so they know what to expect. But it doesn't mean I care more about winning than a lawyer who never sets foot in death row. All it means is I have a different bedside manner. When I'm about to die, I want my doctor to tell me so. I was at the prison seeing Starret so I wouldn't be compelled to see myself as a hypocrite.

Of course, asking a crazy person whether he is comfortable with your plan couldn't make less sense. I might as well have asked him how he'd like a trip to Cancún.

Starret was fifty-four hours from being dead. If we lost, this would be our final face-to-face conversation. He came into the cage on his toes and smiling. He said, What's up, Professor? But then he looked at me, and the smile went away.

I told him I was there because I needed to know whether he wanted us to do anything besides trying to reinstate his appeals. He tilted his head and used his left hand to massage his right wrist. I could see a deep groove where the handcuff had been. He leaned toward me, almost like he was praying. He said, They still got those speakers in the walls, you feel me?

I said, I'm working on that. What I need to know now is whether you want me to pursue legal claims I think are worth pursuing.

He sat back and nearly toppled from the stool. He opened his eyes wide and pursed his lips like he was about to say something, but then he closed his mouth and listed to the left, regaining his balance. He stroked his clean-shaven chin like he had a goatee. He said, I already told you I don't know who that doctor was. Last night they didn't hardly put no corn on my tray. Miss Cara promised she'd get my momma to come see me. I ain't seen her in twenty years, something like that.

I said, Listen, Starret. Here's what I need to know. If I think there is something we can do to try to save your life, do you want us to do it?

He looked at me like he was staring at the quadratic formula. He said, To save my life? Like what? He rubbed his wrist again for half a minute and I thought maybe he had forgotten what I asked. He said, Course I do.

I said, That's what I needed to know.

I spent a few minutes telling him it would probably come down to the wire. They'd take him to the Walls Unit Wednesday around noon and put him in the holding cell adjacent to the execution chamber. I told him Cara or I would come see him there if we had time, but that we probably would not know for sure whether the execution would proceed until nearly six. He smiled. He said, I ordered me some fried chicken, pepperoni pizza, French fries, strawberry ice cream, pecan pie, and Dr Pepper. They gonna pass me all that through the bean slot or do they got a table over there? I told him he'd eat it in the holding cell. He said, Tell Miss Cara to bring her camera so she can take a picture of me feasting, feel me?

Back in my car, I called Cara and asked her to read me the petition. It was two o'clock. We had four hours to get it filed. She had done a terrific job writing up the claim, but there was a big problem. Under state law, once a death row inmate has already gone through the habeas process, he cannot file another habeas appeal unless he satisfies very narrow exceptions. I did not think we had done a good job of explaining why we had met the exception. And the further problem was that if we filed what we had written, and the court concluded we had not satisfied the exception, and we then tried to address that concern and file it again, the court would rule against us unless we could also explain why we had not addressed that concern in what we had already filed. In other words, without being overly technical here, if we screwed up what we were about to file, it would be impossible to fix. I suppose there is always a trade-off between perfection and alacrity, but the price we'd pay for striking the wrong balance would be Starret's life. I said, The Section 5 argument needs to be stronger. I'll work on it when I get to the office.

Cara said, We won't make it by six.

I said, If we file it tomorrow, we might get disbarred. If we file it today, Starret gets executed. I think we have to risk it.

She said, Me too.

■ ■ ■

talk to dead people. They live in my backyard, in the curly willow that started as a stick Katya brought home from her parents' house ten years ago and stuck in the ground next to our pool. Now that tree spreads shade over an area half as big as a tennis court.

At three in the morning on summer nights, when the full moon is low in the west and a southerly breeze blows in from the gulf, the tree's shadow dances on the chair where I sit and sip bourbon on ice while I wait for the dog. That's when they visit. That's how I learned that whether you are dead after you die depends on what you did while you were alive.

Gilbert had a secret someone else revealed to me. He had AIDS. He and his wife had two children and attended service every Sunday at the First Baptist Church until the kids went off to college and Gilbert decided he couldn't keep living a lie. He told his wife and kids one Sunday supper after church, and they hugged him and said they thought so. He and his wife remained friends until he died, and he never stopped being a father to his children or a grandfather to theirs. In a building full of saints, he was still the kindest person in the room. When I asked him one morning how he was doing, he said, What do you know? I told him I didn't know anything, I always ask how he's doing. He said, Yes, but this morning you mean it.

He was the second best pianist to come out of North Texas, right after Van Cliburn. He looked like Van Cliburn, too, all sharp and angular, like he'd stepped off Picasso's easel. One day we were having a drink at Leon's. He said, You know, if I had been born in New York, I would have been perfectly normal. I asked him whether he meant *ordinary*. He said, No. I mean normal.

Gil lives in the tree. Two nights before the Starret execution he said, No queer in America has it harder than an inner-city black man who's gay. I'm from a one-light cattle town full of rednecks and double-wides. I can say that.

Was Starret gay? Did it matter? Was there some legal claim based on that fact I could construct in the remaining hours? I said, What are you saying, Gilbert?, but he was already gone.

Gil and I shared a secretary with Dan. If you wrote a brilliant answer on Dan's exam, you got an A. Everyone else got a C. Nobody had written a brilliant answer in fifteen years. The students called him C-plus Dan. They meant it as a term of affection. Even the GPA-obsessed law review students kept taking his courses.

Dan used to carry a copy of Harry Frankfurt's essay *On Bullshit* in his blazer's inside pocket. I doubt he made small talk even when he talked in his sleep. Most mornings Dan would be leaving the office when I was arriving. We were friends, but if he felt like he had nothing to say, all he'd do was nod hello when our paths crossed in the morning as the sun was rising over Houston's Third Ward.

I once asked him his advice on how to deal with a colleague who wouldn't talk to women and who went to the bathroom to wash after shaking hands with a black man. He told me, You can't always choose who sits down next to you in the lunchroom. I looked at him uncomprehendingly, so he finished the thought. He said, But you can decide how long you stay.

Dan lives there too, on the branch above Gil. He said, You are going to stir up some trouble for yourself, but you won't back down, I know that. You won't disappoint me.

I had no idea what he was talking about. I rubbed my eyes and lay back on the chaise, balancing the tumbler on my chest.

Two days earlier I had taken Winona to our regular vet. The vet wasn't convinced Metacam had caused the problem. She believes in coincidence, but she didn't try to persuade me to start it again. I said, If it wasn't the medicine, what do you think it was?

She said, I don't know.

One thing was clear: Now that Winona was off the drug, she was in pain again. Her gait was stiff and her appetite slight. When she would go outside to relieve herself she would immediately come back in. At bedtime each night I carried her up the stairs.

I fell asleep and dreamed Lincoln was riding her like a horse, screaming with glee. Suddenly she collapsed beneath him. He tried to lift her up but couldn't. He was repeating her name, saying *Nonie, Nonie, get up*, and calling to me for help. I couldn't tell whose eyes showed greater fear.

I didn't hear her stumble downstairs and come outside. She licked my ear and I bolted upright, splashing most of the bourbon onto the ground. I massaged her snout and touched her belly. It still seemed large, but I was relieved to see her standing there. I asked, Are you better? Then I turned and looked again at the tree. I might have gasped. I pointed and said, Look at that, podjo.

Pam was sitting there, right next to where Dan had been. Thirty-five years earlier she'd been my first date. We sat next to each other in AP English and AP math. When I asked her if she would go with me to the seventh-grade formal, she said, I suppose.

I wore a gray suede tuxedo. She wore a red velvet gown. She was the first girl, maybe even the first person, I found intimidating. I had bought her a corsage but my hands were shaking too hard to pin it to her dress, so she took it from me and did it herself. She had said, It is lovely. In my yearbook she wrote, *It's nice to be important, but it's more important to be nice.*

She and her husband had two children. When the kids reached middle school, she left the family retail business and went to law school. She came by my office the day her constitutional law class had discussed *Roe v. Wade*. She said, I don't think I can be a lawyer. I asked her why. She said, I just think there are so many decisions that should be left to individuals to make for themselves, but the law keeps intruding. How can the law not respect human beings to make decisions for themselves?

A month later her neurologist found a brain tumor. He told her she might have three months. She quit law school and hung on for four more years. I flew back to Texas from Utah to go to her funeral. Her kids were there, all grown up. I thought to myself, She stayed until they didn't need her anymore.

I hadn't known she lived in that tree. She said, What I miss terribly is my children. It's really the only thing.

She seemed unbearably sad, or maybe it was me, and then she was gone.

I carried Winona and what was left of my drink upstairs. I sat on the edge of Lincoln's bed and watched him sleep. A month earlier, after a difficult case, I told him at breakfast I was thinking I might stop being a death penalty lawyer. He said, Dada, I don't think you should do that.

When I got to the office the next morning Jeffrey and Cara were finishing up the appeal. They handed it to me to read and I said, I think Starret might have been sexually abused, maybe by his mom, or maybe by kids in his neighborhood.

Jeffrey said, What? When?

Cara said, Why do you all of a sudden think that?

I said, If we get a stay, I think we need to spend a lot of energy looking for evidence of abuse. It's just a feeling I have.

But it never came to that. We got the Starret papers filed by mid-morning. At the end of that day, the state court ruled against us. We stayed up all night and filed an appeal in the Supreme Court first thing Wednesday morning. The clerk called at five thirty to tell me we had lost.

I called Starret. He did not thank me. He said, But I changed my mind. I thought y'all were gonna help me. You promised me. Miss Cara told me we was gonna win.

I heard him muttering. I was not sure if he was talking to himself, to me, or to a guard. I could not understand him. He said, You said you was gonna help. I want my appeal. I didn't get to have my appeal. I didn't get my appeal, man.

I told him I was sorry, but I don't think he heard me. I said, Starret? But he didn't answer. I held the phone to my ear until a guard pulled the receiver away from Starret and placed it in the cradle while my client still pled. Less than thirty minutes later, he was dead.

When Cara got back from the prison, she, Jeffrey, and I walked to the bar next door. Cara said, When I saw him at three he had all that food spread across the bunk in his cell. He asked me whether he'd still get dinner when they took him back to Polunsky.

I asked her how she answered. She said, I told him we needed to hope he'd make it back to the row.

I said, And?

Cara said, He said, Don't you worry none. I'll be back. The professor told me so, you feel me?

I bought us three rounds of drinks. The TV above the bar was showing a replay of the third Ali–Norton fight. I said, Watch this, Ali wins the decision but Norton won the fight.

Cara and Jeffrey looked up at the TV. Neither had yet been born when the fight happened live. Jeffrey said, Are you okay to drive?

I said, I'm fine. It's a metaphor.

I left the two of them sitting there and went home to read Lincoln a story before he went to sleep, but I got there too late. Katya said, He was tired but asked if you would wake him up to say good night. So I went upstairs, and I did.

Thursday morning a sheriff's deputy walked into my office at nine. He handed me a legal document called a show cause order. The Texas court was demanding Cara and I appear before them and explain why we waited so long to try to block the Starret execution. The document listed the punishments we'd face if they did not accept our explanation. Cara said, I don't want to get disbarred.

I said, Might not be so bad.

■ ■ ■

A t the pistol range I used to go to west of Hobby Airport, they called me Grudge because I pinned Polaroids of people I don't like to the targets I'd shoot at from twenty-five meters. I owned four handguns, a bolt-action rifle, and a shotgun. When Lincoln was born Katya wanted me to get rid of them. I asked a friend with a gun safe to store the handguns, and I gave him the rifle in return. But I kept the shotgun. I've got a family to take care of. If anyone ever climbs our stairs at night and doesn't turn and run when he hears the *whoosh* of the pump chambering a shell, I'll know that if the dog doesn't kill him I'm going to have to.

It's important to understand that people who defend murderers aren't necessarily opposed to killing. I work with a decorated veteran who served two tours in a marine infantry unit in Vietnam, and he didn't turn into a liberal when he got home. I work with a Black-hawk helicopter pilot who thinks it was a good idea to invade Iraq even if Saddam Hussein never even wanted weapons of mass destruction. Most of our problems do not result from the fact people disagree. They result because people think they know what someone else thinks about something because of what he thinks about something else.

Two days after I had knee surgery, my assistant asked me how I was doing. I said, We have two lawyers in the office who are dealing with thyroid cancer, one who is battling breast cancer, an investigator who is getting treatment for ovarian cancer, and a paralegal with lymphoma. We don't need smoke alarms here; we need fucking Geiger counters. Thanks for asking, but my knee is irrelevant.

She said, One thing I learned in social work school is that you can't compare pain. Everyone's pain is his own.

I said, See there. That's why I think social work school is a crock. I don't need to experience a double mastectomy to know I'd rather have a torn meniscus.

Experience is nice to have, but it's no substitute for imagination.

■ ■ ■

drove out to the range. Jerry said, Been a while. Thought you'd died, Grudge.

I asked him if I could rent a .357. He handed me the gun and said, Just pay for the shells. You want reloads? I told him I wanted two hundred hollow points. He said, You're gonna waste hollow points on paper targets?

I'd made ten copies of a picture of the state's judges. I'd cut out the few judges I respected. I covered the remaining faces with cartoon characters I got from the morning paper. I wanted to make sure I wasn't violating any laws. I put on a pair of ear protectors, turned 30 degrees away from the targets, and shot for half an hour. When I came back into the shop from the range Jerry was sitting at the counter cleaning the parts of a disassembled .45. He said, Feel better now?

I said, As a matter of fact, I do.

I checked my email in the car. The clerk from the court of appeals had written to ask when we would be filing something for Waterman. The state court had confirmed the date and time of our contempt hearing. There was a surfer alert telling me a late-season storm in the gulf was kicking up six-foot waves. That's as good as it gets in Galveston.

I called Katya and told her I was going to go get wet, but that I'd be home in time to fix dinner. Thirty minutes later I was sitting in my kayak. The ocean was empty as far as I could see, except for two other surfers, who looked like they were skipping eleventh grade. A stiff wind blowing in from the north was keeping the waves glassy and clean. The two surfers and I shared them until the sun was low and my shoulders ached. I waved good-bye and pointed my boat toward shore. But I got too perpendicular to a wave. I slid off the face and the wave stood my kayak straight up until the bow burrowed into the sandy bottom. I leaned forward and kissed the deck as I flipped. The wave broke on top of my upside-down boat, and I would have sworn a trout swam right into my head. I waited until I washed out of the turbulence then rolled back up and spit out a mouth of seawater. I felt great. I laughed out loud and let the swells push me back to the empty beach.

When I got home Katya and Lincoln were playing a duet for piano and flute. I kissed them both then listened to them play while I cooked redfish beignets and a pot of black beans for Katya and me, and a bowl of pasta for our vegetarian son. Over dinner I told them about the show cause order. I never get mad because Katya gets mad enough for both of us. Where I see idiots and react with amusement, she sees evil and responds with passion. She kept saying Unbelievable. Unfucking believable.

I smiled and said, Hey, watch your language in front of our son.

She said, It's appropriate for the context.

Lincoln said, I don't understand. Are they going to punish you for trying to help someone?

I kissed him on the head and said to Katya, What a guy.

illy Parham in The Crossing *is the opposite of me. He is the anti-metaphysician. All he does is act. There is logic and beauty and truth to his actions, but they are not entailed by any obvious or articulable philosophy. You want me to be Billy Parham, but I cannot. I am a man who stews.*

Inaction is not always a sign of weakness. It can be an emblem of strength. It can be a statement of character. We've talked before about what you would do if you were one of your clients, whether you would say good-bye to everyone you know or spend all your time with those you love the most; whether you would try new foods or eat your old favorites; whether you would read new books or reread passages of those you treasure most.

That's what we have talked about when we have talked about you, because you think you need answers to those questions. I do not. I think the question is enough. Maybe you won't eat at all, but instead just contemplate the alternatives. Then you need not choose.

Sometimes when I finish a wonderful book I do not immediately return it to the shelf and begin something new. Sometimes I just turn back through what I have finished, rereading some passages, some entire pages. I might just sit there holding the book, turning it in my hands, not thinking about anything I could verbalize, but simply experiencing the sensation of having finished a beautiful book. Don't you at times listen to a piece of music and remain in the rapture even after the CD ends?

I am no longer reading, but I am still savoring the experience. I am in fact doing something. Don't you ever just sit there and enjoy?

What I am trying to say is that I might not be moving, I might not be doing anything, but I am not passive. I am living the way I want to be living, given my capabilities.

Tomorrow they cut open my skull. So this might be the last letter I ever write. If it is, you will honor me by turning it over in your hands.

■　■　■

One night during my third year of law school, my best friend Jon and I were eating huge plates of eggplant parmigiana at Biagetti's in North Haven and drinking cheap red wine from a gallon jug. There was the sound of gunfire from the street, and two guys wearing suits eating at the table next to ours went running outside, pulling snub-nosed revolvers from the small of their backs as they went. I said to Jon, I think maybe I'll interview with the FBI.

He rolled his eyes and said, You do that.

I said, What's wrong with the idea?

He said, Dow, in case you haven't noticed, you have problems with authority. You wouldn't last a day.

I said, I do not have a problem with authority. I have a problem with idiots.

He said, Distinction without a difference. You think anyone who doesn't agree with you is an idiot.

I met Cara and Maurice at the court. There's an old joke: Any attorney who represents himself has a fool for a client. The judges came out. They seemed surprised to see three people instead of only two. One asked, You're represented by counsel? I thought to myself, Yes we are, you idiot.

Maurice stood, introduced himself as our lawyer, and walked to the podium. He was there to explain how we had three choices: We could have filed nothing, we could have filed the petition outside the forty-eight-hour window, or we could have done what we did. He quickly dismissed the first option. We were Starret's lawyers. Our legal and ethical obligation was to represent him zealously, within the bounds of the law. Once we identified what we believed was a compelling legal claim, we were bound to pursue it. That left the remaining two options. Maurice explained the obvious. Texas law is unforgiving to death row inmates who file a habeas petition and then want to make it better by elaborating on an argument in that petition. In some states, and in federal court, it is possible to amend a habeas petition and articulate points that fell through the cracks when the petition was originally filed. The Texas court, however, regularly construes a supplemental or amended petition as an entirely new petition. The reason this is a problem is that the law places severe limitations on when a new petition can be filed. In short, if we had hurriedly filed the petition outside the forty-eight-hour period, and then sought to supplement the petition the next day, the court would have deemed the supplement a new petition, and we would have been barred from filing it on the grounds we should have included the argument in our original filing.

Maurice was just telling them what they already knew, daring them to argue. Not a single judge did. Instead, they wanted to ask him about the merits of the claim we were raising. Maurice said he thought I was the better person to answer those questions, so I replaced him at the podium. For nearly half an hour, the judges peppered me with questions about the *Batson* claim. They wondered why I thought we had a claim at all. A version of the claim had been raised during a previous appeal and they asked why I thought I could raise it again. We discussed the similarities between my case and another case where the court had permitted a lawyer representing a death row inmate to do just what I had done. Not a single judge asked me about timing. No one asked what had prevented me from getting it filed the day before.

I sat down and Cara stood up. Earlier, when we arrived at the courthouse, she had signed an exact copy of the statement I had written and given it to the clerk. She told the judges she had done so, and asked whether anyone had questions for her. No one did. She sat down thirty seconds after she rose.

On the way back to Houston Cara and I made a bet. I told her we would never hear from the court again. I said, There is no way they can conclude we waited too long because they did not ask me even a single question about timing. If they are going to criticize us for not filing a day earlier, wouldn't they have to ask at least one question about why we did not file a day earlier so they could deem that explanation unsatisfactory? And yet there is not a chance in hell they are going to write an opinion saying I did nothing wrong. All that leaves them with is silence.

I said, I'll bet you a dollar we hear nothing further.

Cara said, You're on.

Five months later, when we had yet to hear a word, Cara conceded. At our biweekly team meeting, she presented me with a dollar.

Two months after that, we received an order from the court. The judges rejected my explanation. Even though they had asked me no questions, they ruled my answers unsatisfactory. They held I violated the forty-eight-hour rule. They let me off with a warning, but stated if it happened again, the consequences would be severe. They said they might bar me from appearing before them anymore.

Cara, of course, had done exactly the same thing I did. Her written statement was identical to mine. They dismissed the charges against her.

At our next meeting, I gave her two dollars. She framed one of them and hung it on her office wall.

■ ■ ■

I tried to kill myself last night.

I took out the windsurfer at dusk. I had not eaten all day because the surgery is this morning. Irmi asked me not to go. I told her I would be fine. I said it might be my last time on the water. There was no kindness in my voice.

The lake is low. I hit a stump I did not see and fell. I sat there, straddling the board. Maybe I was too tired or too weak to hoist the sail out of the water, maybe I just thought I was. It doesn't matter. Although it is possible to have strength in reserve even if one believes the tank to be empty, it is also possible to be wrong. So I just sat bobbing, calculating where on the shoreline the lake's ululations would take me. The thought that Irmi would think I had drowned entered my brain unbidden, and so it was suddenly obvious that I should drown. It is a frightful death only to those who struggle against it, and I did not intend to struggle.

I slipped off the board, exhaling, kicking off my surf shoes, feeling the water grow colder as I sank. I felt my toes reach the muck. I exhaled all I thought was left of my breath and watched the bubbles rise toward the fading luminescence. I folded myself over to press out the last of the air and congratulated myself for being so clever. Irmi would get the insurance money, because it could have been an accident. Of course it could. Even strong men die windsurfing.

175

And then I was aware I needed a breath. I was aware I was only moments of oxygen deprivation away from unconsciousness, and that suddenly, I did not want to die. I did not want to die away from Irmi.

I had told Irmi we'd barbeque with you and Katya over the weekend. I could not let my final words to her be lies. I was being the opposite of selfless. I know you think this is not unusual, and I am not prepared to argue with you over it, but I was aware of my selfishness, and it displeased me.

My lungs were burning. I could feel cells in my brain clicking off like burned-out lightbulbs. My vision began to darken.

I bent my knees to push off the bottom toward the top, and I pushed as hard as I could. I sank deeper down into the muck. The panic was entirely gone, and I was simply sad. Involuntarily I started to breathe. I gagged and swallowed water. I hoped I didn't remain at the bottom of this lake. I hoped Irmi would find me. My last wish was for her. That thought rescued me.

Finally my feet popped loose, and I sprinted a breaststroke upward, sucking in air at the exact moment I broke through the surface. I saw my board just ten meters away, but I had no interest in retrieving it. I rolled onto my back, breathing between coughs, and frog-kicked toward shore. I was not happy to be alive. I was relieved not to be dead. I did not want to be gone before telling you and Katya and Philip and Irmi, mostly Irmi, good-bye.

Richter tells a story about one of his teachers, Heinrich Neuhaus. They worked together on the Liszt B Minor Sonata. Richter says Neuhaus taught him the importance of the silences, but it was Richter who took the lesson to an extreme. He would come out onstage and sit down at the piano, and he would play nothing. The first note is a G. Richter calls it a miserable G sound. He would sit on the bench, eyes straight ahead, and slowly count to thirty. Richter says he could feel the audience, feel them fidgeting, squirming, wondering. Until finally, he would play the G, now unexpected, now a relief, and hence no longer miserable.

These treatments are making me into the expectant audience. They're the silence. The rest of my life is that miserable G, but it is less miserable than this. Once they've cut open my skull and dug through my brain, the music begins. I am through with the doctors. I am moving on with what is left.

■ ■ ■

I didn't fall in love with Katya the first time I saw her.

It was the third time. We went to see *Jacob's Dream* at the old Tower theater then had drinks at Bitterman's and stayed there talking until they closed. She told me about a young girl named Lori she was mentoring through the Big Brothers Big Sisters program. I said, It's dangerous for you to drive into that neighborhood by yourself.

She said, No it isn't. Everyone on the street knows why I'm there.

I said, It doesn't matter. You should carry a can of Mace.

She said, You can trust people or not trust them. Either way you'll be wrong sometimes. I'd rather be wrong trusting.

I drove us back to my house. We sat on the sofa in my library listening to Lester Young and Oscar Peterson. Whitney, my first Doberman, flopped down between us, her head on Katya's thigh. We talked all night. She said, Every time I drive up to Lori's house I get depressed, and by the time I leave I'm happy. She gives me as much as I give her.

When the sun came up I made French toast from stale challah and strong coffee for breakfast. Katya took a swallow and said, Do you have any milk? I didn't. I had used it all up for the egg wash. She said, How about ice cream?

Her mom thought Katya was wasting her time with me. I was in my thirties, obsessed with my work, and set in my ways. I didn't often think about the distant future, but on the rare occasion when an image of my life thirty years down the road muscled itself into my brain, I didn't see a wife and children. I saw an old man living alone in the country with a dog. One morning, after we'd been seeing each other for four years, I got home after a night of playing cards and Katya was sitting on the bathroom floor next to Whitney, whose spinal cancer made it hard for her to stand. I sat down next to her. She said, I think our time is running out.

She stayed with me until three months later, when Whitney finally died. She was with me at the vet, and for two weeks after, and then one day, as she was leaving for New York for her law firm's annual meeting, she said, I'm going to be moving my things back to my apartment when I get back. I can't do this anymore.

I said, Can't we talk about this?

She said, There isn't any point. I know what you'll say, and I know you love me. You just don't love me the way I need to be loved. She kissed me and got in the car to the airport. Three days later, when I got home from the office, her clothes were gone from the closet.

When Whitney stopped responding to the radiation, when it became clear there wouldn't be a miracle, I asked the vet how I'd know when it was time. He said, You'll know.

I'm not sure he was right. One thing I've learned is that beginnings are unambiguous, but endings are not.

My mother is the eldest of three children. Her father, my Zaide Liebe, said children are like fingers. You love them all the same. Maybe that's true for most parents, but not for me. I read somewhere that Larry Bird didn't get engaged until his Doberman died. Some people have only so much room in their hearts. I left Katya messages and wrote her letters until she finally let me tell her what I had learned about myself. She listened to me intensely, then she said, Here's the problem: The best predictor of future behavior is past conduct.

I said, Yes, but I can change. I've already changed.

She said, Everyone thinks that. You live your life by your rules.

I resorted to platitudes. I said, Rules have exceptions.

She was leaning against a bookshelf, her arms crossed, her mind made up. The sun had set and the room was turning dark. She wasn't going to let herself be hurt.

I said, I figured something out, Katya. The exceptions to your rules are the meaning of love.

My neighbor's car pulled into his drive and the headlights briefly lit the room. I stepped toward her. When I held her, she let me. That night was not the first time I told Katya I loved her. I believe, though, it was the first time she believed me.

Three months later we got Winona. Six months after that I asked Katya to marry me. Her parents were hiking in the interior of Mexico, completely incommunicado. We couldn't talk to them for another week. I was secretly elated. It meant by the time they learned the news it would be too old for them to try to talk Katya out of it. They probably wouldn't have tried anyway, but I didn't want to risk it. I'd used up all my aces.

On our wedding night, at two fifteen, Katya and I said good night to the forty remaining guests who had nowhere else they wanted to be, and we took the elevator to the fourteenth floor. I carried her into the suite. We were laughing and drunk. I remembered our suitcases in the lobby and went back down, kissing Katya before I left, saying I'd be right back. I told everyone good night again.

As I picked up our bags, the hotel's power failed. The only illumination came from the brake lights of cars lined up in the driveway to leave. I asked someone where were the stairs. The hotel's chief engineer saw me stumbling and said, Come with me. We walked through narrow halls like a submarine and came to the freight elevator. He said, Separate power source. Go ahead and get on.

It wobbled as it rose. Last week Lincoln, at the age of nine, told me that elevators have eight cables. There's also a brake. In other words, he said with reassurance, there's plenty of redundancy.

I said, Redundancy?

He said, Yes, Dada. But if they fail anyway, lie down on the floor so you spread your weight around. I told him I wasn't sure that would matter. He laughed and said, Probably not.

The elevator suddenly stopped. After a moment of pure blackness, a single emergency bulb clicked on, like a bomb shelter from *The Road*. The engineer took out his radio. Juan, do you read me? Juan?

Juan didn't answer. The engineer radioed Juan six more times. He couldn't look at me.

Meanwhile, Katya was wandering up and down the darkened hallways calling my name, wondering if she had been right about me all along. I heard her only in my head.

An hour and fifteen minutes later, help arrived. We were stuck between floors three and four. Two mechanics turned a lever and dropped us down to three. The engineer told me to follow him again, and he led us to the stairs. He offered to help with my bags, one holding our clothes, one filled with books, but I wanted to be alone. I carried them up eleven flights. In my heart I already knew as I walked I would never abandon those I love, or those who think they need me. But there, on the landing between floors eleven and twelve, I resolved to make sure they knew it, too.

And suddenly, there was my bride, still wearing her gown, standing next to the elevators, staring up at the unlit panel of numbers. She said, Where have you been?

I said, Long story. Why are you still dressed?

She said, I think I'm stuck.

Her attendants had pinned her dress closed. She couldn't undo them. I held her face in my hands. I said, Katya, you're never getting rid of me.

Her laugh, I think, might have started as a cry.

■ ■ ■

eter's brain surgery lasted three hours. The surgeon came out
and said they had cut out three marble-size tumors. Irmi nodded, saying nothing. Katya asked him whether there were
others they had missed. The surgeon said no. Katya asked him
whether others would grow. The surgeon said to ask the oncologist.
Katya said, You're the one here. I'm asking you. His cheeks turned
red. He said probably so, and he took a step away. I thought of that
children's experiment where kids put similarly charged metal shavings next to each other and watch them repel, and I smiled. The
surgeon became an ostrich, thinking he could avoid danger by avert-
ing his eyes. He turned from Katya and looked directly at Irmi, and
told her Peter would be able to go home in two days.

When I went into the recovery room he was sleeping. I talked to
him anyway.

I said, One thing I've learned is that there is no relationship between what you've done and what you get. Weber's Protestants were
wrong to think there is. The Nazis' victims did not bring it upon
themselves. People who play the lottery and win are no better than
the millions who lose. If you're saying what you're saying about de-
serving this fate out of anger and frustration, I'm fine with it. But
if you believe this nonsense, if you've turned into Pat Robertson,

you're going to force me to embarrass you by cataloguing every act of loving-kindness you've ever performed, and I'm not sure you'll live long enough for me to get to the end.

His eyelids flickered open, then closed again. I think he tried to smile. He mouthed, *Thank you.*

■ ■ ■

On Saturday Peter went home. We went to the lake the next day to visit. Katya had been reading about experimental immunotherapy. Even though they'd lost his liver, Katya wanted her dad to ask the oncologist for some dead melanoma cells, or some antigens from those cells, and have a vaccine made from them. She wanted him to inject that vaccine, in combination with interleukin-2. She said it wouldn't cure him, but it would delay the return of the tumors.

She also wanted him to take vemurafenib. Half the people with melanoma have a mutation in what is called the BRAF gene; that mutation causes the gene to make an altered protein, and that altered protein makes melanoma cells proliferate. Vemurafenib inhibits the activity of the protein or enzyme. Like the immunotherapy, vemurafenib would not cure him, but it would prolong his life by slowing the tumor growth.

He said, *No.*

Katya said, *No? That's all you have to say?*

We don't even know if I have the BRAF mutation, and besides, some people who took the drug developed new cancers. As for the vaccines, Katya, the data give one no reason for hope. I read How We Die. *The author, Sherwin Nuland, had a brother who died of cancer. I do not know what kind. Dr. Nuland says the thing he most regrets was not being able to talk truthfully to his brother about his prognosis. I made a note in the margin where Nuland lamented not saying things he should have said. He should have said them because they were true, and we owe truth to those we love. Nuland examines why he withheld truth, and he concludes it was to avoid causing his brother pain and to give him hope. But Nuland put the word* hope *in quotation marks, and he called it a misconceived hope. As a doctor, Nuland knew there was no hope. The cancer would win. He faults himself for hiding that from his brother. I think we owe each other honesty, liebe.*

Katya said, Western doctors do not believe what they cannot explain. They cannot explain why hope would matter, so they say it isn't true. But our entire existence is ultimately inexplicable. That doesn't mean we do not exist.

Peter smiled. He said, *You've been brainwashed by your husband.*

She said, Oh Papa, and she hugged him. His cheeks looked hollow enough to hold billiard balls.

He said, *Nothing warms the cockles of my heart more than your desire that I live. But the fact you want something is not enough to mend me.* He used his thumb to wipe a tear from Katya's chin. He said, *Liebe, just because life is impossible is no reason not to enjoy it.*

I said, Joyce?

He said, *Close. Svevo.* He looked toward the kitchen then said, *I think Irmi needs you to carve the roast beef. She doesn't trust me with the knife.*

■　■　■

When I got to my office Jeffrey was sitting there with a black woman I didn't know. He introduced her to me. He said, Tamira Sanders is the woman who testified Waterman robbed her at the gas station. I raised my eyebrows. Jeffrey said, In her police report, she said she'd remember the guy who hit her because of his tattoo. Turns out, all the guys in the car had the same tattoo. I showed her a picture of all four taken after the McClain murder. I also played her audiotapes from his testimony at trial. She is positive the one who hit her is Johnston. Positive.

I said to Jeffrey, Ten years ago she was positive it was Waterman.

To her I said, Ms. Sanders, you told police and the jury you'd never forget his voice.

She said, I know. I told the truth. What I remembered when Mr. Jeffrey here came and talked to me is that two of them were talking back and forth. The window on the passenger side was down. I can't say whether the voice I remember came from inside or outside. Anyway, the police told me it was your client who beat me. They already knew.

I said, They told you?

She said, Uh-huh.

I said, Are you telling me you simply agreed with something they told you was true?

187

She said, Yes sir. That's how it was.

I said, Will you sign an affidavit for us?

She said, I ain't going to say I was wrong. Maybe I wasn't. I'm just willing to say I ain't sure no more.

After she signed the statement and was about to leave, she said, In case the TV or newspaper people call me about this, I want you to know I'm not against the death penalty. There's some bad people who don't deserve to be walking God's fine earth.

I said, Ms. Sanders, I agree with you on that. I just don't think the State of Texas should be deciding who those people are. Either way, you should feel free to say whatever you want to the media if they call you. Thank you for your honesty, and your courage.

Jeffrey, Cara, and I sat down with our investigator, two students, and our list of the seven guards we wanted to talk to. Three of them lived in a rural area just south of the prison. The guard whose license plate number I had written down outside Florida's restaurant lived in Woodville, about thirty miles to the east. Two were retired and living in Tyler, and one was a cop in Galveston. I saw a chance to squeeze in a few hours of surfing. I said, I'll take the guy in Galveston, then I'll find my pal from Florida's Restaurant.

I asked Jeffrey to go to Tyler. He said, I think Smith County might have more racists per square inch than anyplace on earth.

I said, Exactly. If you can get those two middle-age white guys to say a black gang member shouldn't be executed, even the Board of Pardons and Paroles should take notice.

He said, Okay, but when I finish with them, I'll take your friend from Florida's. It's an easy trip for me, and it will give me a reason to leave Tyler no matter what time of night I'm done.

I said, Have at it.

That left Cara and two students to talk to the three active guards who lived near their work. I thought they'd be the least likely to help. I said, Be sure to record them. If they get cold feet and decide not to sign statements, we might need proof of what they said, if they say anything good, which I doubt they will.

She asked, Do we tell them we're taping them?

I looked at Jeffrey. He said, It's Texas. We don't have to.

I said, No, I want them to know. Go ahead and conspicuously hit the record button on your iPhone when you're introducing yourself. That ought to be notice enough.

With my kayak on top of my truck, I headed to Galveston. Sergeant Wendell Peterson worked in the jail division of the Galveston County Sheriff's Department, but he'd been a guard for the Texas Department of Criminal Justice for eleven years, including four on death row. He lived in a duplex two blocks off the strand. When I rang the bell, no one answered, so I drove to the jail. The desk sergeant pointed me back to his cubicle. When I introduced myself and said why I was there, he said, I ain't talking about that here. I asked if I could talk to him later, and he told me to meet him at O'Malley's at four.

I spent an hour in the surf and still got to the bar with half an hour to spare. I ordered a double of Jameson neat and the bartender poured me what looked like half a liter. Peterson walked in right on time. He sat down next to me and the bartender poured him a shot and drew him a draft without his saying a word. He said, I heard some judge says Waterman's cousin's a retard.

In fact, the lawyer for Waterman's cousin—the young man whose shot had killed Miss McClain—had persuaded the state court to examine whether his client was mentally retarded, and therefore immune from execution. I said, Not exactly. There's a court looking into it. From what I know, I doubt it will go anywhere.

He drained half his mug. He said, Waterman tell you to come see me? I told him he had. He said, Boy's got him a memory. I told him 'fore I left if I could ever do him some favor, to write me and say so. I asked him why he'd made the offer. He looked at his reflection in the mirror behind the bar, or maybe he was looking back behind him. He said, I ain't opposed to the death penalty, not one bit. Most of them ride the needle would kill you for your shoes.

When you need something from someone is not the time to catalogue your disagreements or disgust with his lazy generalizations. One thing I've learned is not to always speak my mind to strangers. I said, Yep.

He said, I have me a little ranch in Brazoria. Waterman got out, I'd hire him to be my hand, trust him to run the place without me even being there. I ain't saying he should get out. Matter of fact, I don't know what he done. All I know is that boy ain't interested in hurting nobody. He's done grown up.

I asked him whether I could write down what he said and have him sign it. He said, Course. DA here in Galveston County don't send no one to the row. They won't care what I say.

The bartender had poured him another shot and another beer. My glass was half full. I pulled a laptop out of my bag while Sergeant Peterson talked to a man no more than three feet tall wearing seersucker shorts, a long-sleeve plaid shirt buttoned up to his neck, red suspenders, and a porkpie hat. I finished the affidavit and waited for the short man to leave. Sergeant Peterson saw me staring. He said, That's Benny. Might not look it, but I swear he's the best fishing guide on this island. You want to catch redfish, he's who you call. I said I just might. He said, Lots a guys' looks can be deceiving, ain't that right?

Sergeant Peterson read what I wrote and said, Yes sir. That's pretty much how I said it. I asked him whether there was anything he wanted to add or change. He said, Nope. I printed the two-page statement on my portable printer and handed him a pen.

One down, six to go.

■ ■ ■

When I was in seventh grade I wanted to run the 400 meters. (Back then it was the 440.) In practice I kept finishing last. It wasn't from lack of effort. I threw up after every race. One day the coach said to me, Dow, you gotta have chicken to make chicken salad.

One thing I've learned is that truth can sting, but it can't actually hurt you. I never did make the team, but I tried. What I lack in talent I try to make up for with will. So for my fiftieth birthday, I decided to run a marathon. I hate running long distances. Anybody can do something they love.

As part of my preparation, I ran a half marathon. Katya and Lincoln were going to run the 5K. The night before, the three of us checked into a hotel a block from the starting line, walked across the street to pick up our registration packets, then settled in to our room. I turned on the Cowboys game. My phone rang. Cara said, The students got arrested. They're in the Polk County jail. What do you want me to do?

They had taken two cars to a community south of Livingston. Cara went searching for the female, whose address we were unsure of, and directed the students to talk to the two young males, who happened to be brothers. They lived in separate trailer homes on a five-acre tract two miles south of the prison. Cara drove into town, if you can call a collection of chain stores and fast-food joints a town, and searched for Officer Morgan. The students drove to the acreage.

One hundred feet up a rutted dirt driveway was a rust-stained mobile home with a sagging deck and an above-ground pool. Two dogs were drinking from the oil-sheened water. The students climbed four wooden steps and knocked on the screen door. A middle-age white woman smoking a menthol cigarette opened the door and said, What ch'all sellin'? The students explained why they were there, that they worked for me, and whom they were there to see. The woman said, Pete 'n Charlie are my boys. Pete lives in the first home, 'bout fifty yards past the storage shed, on the right. Charlie's where the road ends. Charlie might still be sleepin', but I know Pete's up. I just done talked to him. Y'all go on ahead and drive on back. The dogs won't bother you none. They're all bark. All bark. Y'all hear that, Laurel and Hardy? The dogs, which had lain down on their sides, lifted their heads. The students said thank you and turned.

Pete was waiting for them, standing in his doorway, wearing his uniform. He walked down three cinder-block steps but didn't offer to shake hands. The students repeated what they'd told his mom. Pete's eyes darted back toward the road. He rubbed the back of his hand across his mouth. He looked nervous and said, I don't know. Y'all shouldn't a come out here. He glanced up toward Charlie's house and then back down toward his mom's. He said, I ain't sure it's a good idea for me to be a talkin' to y'all. Who'd y'all say yer working for?

The students told him they were just trying to get some insight from some of the guards on the row into how Waterman had changed. They said, We already talked to a couple. It was their only lie. Pete asked them who.

Charlie walked up, trailed by two bird dogs. He said, Who's your company, Pete? Pete told him. Charlie said, Aw man. He faced the students. He said, Waterman's about the last man there should be gettin' the juice. Pete looked at him. Charlie said, Shit, Pete. They cain't fire me for saying what's on my mind when I ain't even on the job. Charlie looked at the students and said, They cain't, can they? The students said they weren't sure, it might depend on whether he had signed any agreements. But they weren't lawyers, they said, just second-year law students.

Pete said, They're just a couple a law students, Charlie, from New York City or some shit.

Charlie said, Well, I ain't gonna sign nothin' anyway but I told you what I think.

Pete said, I don't want to be rude or nothin' but I'm gonna ask y'all to go now. Charlie shrugged his shoulders but didn't argue. The students thanked the men for their time.

They sat in the car for a minute or two more typing notes onto their laptops. Then they made a four-point turn at the end of the road, right in front of Charlie's house, and headed nose first back down the drive. They stopped at the blacktop, put on the turn signal, and looked both ways. As soon as they turned onto the highway, a sheriff's deputy turned on his flashing lights and pulled them over.

I had just opened a beer and plopped down on the bed, wearing sweats, and elevated my legs. My pre–run day ritual. Katya and Lincoln had ordered room service. On the TV, which I had muted, Jerry Jones was screaming at somebody about something. I did not want to go down to the garage, collect my car, and drive to Polk County. I said, Shit, Cara, I have a race tomorrow morning.

She said, They're probably freaking out.

I said, I doubt anything bad will happen to them in the county jail. It's not like they have a bunch of gangbangers in Polk County. Let 'em have some dinner and a good night's sleep. I'll drive up tomorrow afternoon and get them out. Cara said nothing. I said, I'm kidding for God's sake.

She said, I knew that.

She was calling from the jail's parking lot. I asked her to go inside and wing it. I asked her to drop her phone into her purse without breaking the connection so I could listen in. I told her if things went south I'd call a judge at home and get an order to release them, and her too, if it came to that.

It didn't. Cara walked in and demanded to see the ranking officer. The desk sergeant pointed her back to the lieutenant's office. Without taking his feet off his desk, the lieutenant leered at her. I know this because I heard Cara say, I know your boss. I go drinking with him. Keep your eyes above my neck, pissant.

I heard the man say, What the, but Cara cut him off. She told him she represented the two students and wanted to see them right away. She demanded to know what they were being charged with and wanted to see a copy of the offense report. She said she was on her way to a judge's house to get him to release them but wanted to be able to tell him what kind of trumped-up charge the sheriff had filed. I heard the lieutenant say, Just a minute. I heard him mutter *bitch* in a stage whisper. Then I heard the sound of a door closing.

Cara took the phone out of her purse and said, He just closed me in his office. Either I'll be leaving here soon with them, or you're going to have to ruin your day.

It was Option A. The lieutenant returned three minutes later with two nervous up-and-coming lawyers trailing behind him. He said, I'm gonna let these two off with a warning. Happens again, I ain't gonna be as forgiving next time. I could practically hear Cara roll her eyes. I heard her say, Thank you, Lieutenant. She's learned, too, to hold her peace.

Cara took the two of them to an icehouse across the county line and bought them Cokes. She drank a beer. They were back in Houston in less than two hours.

Later we learned that when Pete saw them sitting in their car with laptops, he got nervous and called his boss at the prison. His boss shared an apartment with a sheriff's deputy. He called the deputy and asked him to pick up the kids. The deputy had laughed and said, Couple a East Coast liberals in the county lockup? Sounds like fun.

The guards didn't give us affidavits, but it didn't matter. My students didn't have to spend a night in jail. One out of two is as good as it gets in my line of work.

■ ■ ■

A dry cold front was blowing in and Lincoln asked me to light a fire. Winona was standing by the back door. I said, While I'm getting the wood, can you take Winona outside?

Through the kitchen window I watched them. Squirrels were scampering around the yard, but Winona paid them no mind. The sky looked like a charcoal drawing with streaks of red. Winona knelt to drink from the pool. I watched her collapse and fall onto the top step.

Lincoln screamed, *Nonie,* and started to cry. I rushed outside and pulled her out. Her pupils were the size of pinpricks. She was inert in my arms. Katya came running with a towel. We called our vet and she sent us straight to the dog ER.

Winona was responsive but unable to stand. Her belly was huge. She winced when the doctor touched it. A technician inserted an IV and drew blood. The doctor said, She is bleeding again, but I am not sure from where. We'll need to sedate her and do a CT scan. She might be having liver failure but I won't know until we get the results of the blood work.

I said, When will that be?

He said, Tomorrow.

He knew we didn't want to go. He said, You have to leave her here. I will call you as soon as we know something.

I picked up Lincoln, and Katya and I held hands. I have no recollection of driving home. Katya took Lincoln upstairs while I picked up the logs I had dropped on the kitchen floor. She put him in our bed, and the two of us sat there in silence until he fell asleep. I walked downstairs and had a drink, then I poured myself another.

It was the first night Winona spent away from us and out of our house in more than thirteen years.

■ ■ ■

Three days before Waterman's execution we assembled in the conference room at seven. There were two slices left from the pizza Cara and the students had shared the night before. Jeffrey came in with a box of donuts and ate one of the slices. I said, I might need to pay you more, partner.

We had the affidavit I'd gotten in Galveston, an affidavit from the interns, reporting what Charlie had said, and an affidavit from a guard at the unit Cara had gotten before the students went to jail. Best of all, even though the guards in Tyler said nothing except no comment, Jeffrey had found the captain whose license plate number I had copied at Florida's. He was eating dinner with his wife and two children at the Cracker Barrel. Jeffrey sat in a booth and nursed a cup of coffee until they finished, then followed them outside. He quickly introduced himself to the captain and said why he was there. The captain said, You have a car? When Jeffrey said he did, the captain said, Follow me.

Once his family went inside he sat in Jeffrey's car in his driveway for more than an hour. His affidavit ran to nearly five single-spaced pages. He said he'd known Waterman since the day he arrived on death row. He said he had never seen an inmate, on death row or otherwise, mature so much so quickly. He said Waterman kept guards from getting shanked. He said Waterman could get through to even the most incorrigible prisoners. He said Waterman was getting his GED and even taking college courses. He said Waterman had taught himself chess and organized a daily discussion group where guys talked about the people they'd injured and why. He said he's a death penalty supporter and a Christian, and there was no way his God would think any good would come from killing Waterman. Jeffrey said the captain started to cry three different times.

Jeffrey smiled. It was possibly the third time I saw him smile in the six years I've known him. He said, Clemency or successor?

A clemency petition is a request that an inmate's life be spared. We had already filed one for Waterman, but Jeffrey was suggesting we supplement it. Clemency requests go to seven people who make up the Board of Pardons and Paroles. They are appointed by the governor. In my experience, most of them are about as open-minded as the Taliban. Somebody on death row could morph into Mother Teresa herself, and those seven people would say, Too bad. She shouldn't have killed anybody. Off with her head.

In other words, clemency petitions are a useless sacrifice of a tree. On the other hand, the argument we were making—that Waterman was remorseful, repentant, and literally a changed man—was a moral argument, not really a legal argument. And that's what the clemency process is designed for. A successor, in contrast, is a legal argument, and we'd be making that argument in a state court, the Texas Court of Criminal Appeals, filled with nine judges most of whom think their job is to make the appellate process faster, not fairer. Plus which, I couldn't even think of a way to package the moral facts into a legal argument. Jeffrey said, What if we argue Waterman is no longer a future danger and therefore not eligible for death?

I said, I like it.

As I've said, defendants in Texas get sentenced to death if the jury decides at their trial that they will be dangerous in the future. Under Texas law, death row inmates can go back to court, can file what is called a successive appeal, if they can point to new facts they could not have discovered previously. Jeffrey was suggesting that the new fact was Waterman's very essence. It could not have been previously discovered because it did not exist at the time of his trial, or even at the time of his original appeal. And, the argument continued, if the jury had known then what we know now about Waterman, it would never have sentenced him to death.

Cara said, Plus, if we get denied, maybe the Supremes will be interested.

When a death row inmate returns to state court, there are basically two ways he can lose. One is for the court to address the merits of the argument and rule against him. The other is for the court to say the inmate is not allowed to come back. If the court uses this latter approach, then it is for all intents and purposes impossible to get the Supreme Court interested in the case, because the justices rarely review a state court's procedural rulings. Our only real hope was for the state court to bite and say our legal argument was unsound.

But one thing I've learned is that there are two kinds of judges in the world, and contrary to what you might have heard from bloviating politicians and pundits, the difference is not between judges who make the law versus judges who interpret the law. All judges interpret. The difference is between the judges whose interpretations agree with yours, and those whose don't. Unfortunately for us, and of course for Waterman, the state court judges were pretty much just like Judge Norton, the federal judge. They believed someone who said *That's how you smoke a bitch* should be executed, and they'd do whatever they had to do to achieve their desire, even if it meant twisting or ignoring the law.

I said, I doubt the CCA will help us out with a decision on the merits. Just because they're dark-hearted and not terribly bright doesn't mean they're stupid. They know how to insulate their decisions from Supreme Court review if they want to.

Jeffrey said, That's true. But the Supreme Court can see through them.

He wasn't smiling anymore, but I was. I love working with these two. I looked at them both and said, The two of you can arm wrestle over who gets to keep Pollyanna as a nickname. Let's file both. It's only paper.

■ ■ ■

eter's hair had already grown back over the spot where doctors had cut out a postage stamp–size piece of his skull so they could scoop out part of his brain. He was holding a book of Richard Feynman lectures in his lap, but he was not reading. He was listening to Horowitz play Mozart's B Minor adagio. His eyes were closed. He said, *Kierkegaard said when we take pleasure in this music we celebrate Mozart's suffering. If beauty comes from suffering, does that make the suffering worthwhile?*

I said, No.

He said, *I am less certain than you.*

I said, As always.

He smiled. He said, *It's because I am not so bothered as you by mysteries.* He touched the book and said, *Feynman says that at a deep stage, the explanations must end. We get to a point where we cannot know any more.*

I said, A hundred years ago Kelvin said we knew everything except a few details. Probably every physicist who's ever lived thinks that.

Peter said, *A year ago I read a paper arguing that elementary particles are really tiny strings vibrating in eleven-dimensional space. I wondered what that means. Last night I was thinking how my genetic ancestors were dying in Africa seven million years ago, seven million years, and it made me wonder why I would ever have cared about understanding eleven dimensions. What relationship does that question have to matters of importance?*

He picked up the remote control and turned up the volume. He said, *Listen here how much faster Horowitz plays it than Brendel.* His eyes were open now. They looked milky and tired. He had lost much of his hair, but his eyebrows were still thick and full. I could see a pulse in the soft flesh beneath his left eye. At that moment I saw Peter for the first time as an old man, and as I did I felt myself grow older, too.

He said, *I do not care if Feynman was right about physics, but I do not think he was right about love.*

We sat there until the music ended and the disc started again. Peter turned down the volume. He said, *I do not know whether I would have suffered had I made other choices at diverging nodes on my life's flow chart, but now I think my choices were overly influenced by the very possibility of suffering. I fear I made wrong choices. In every endeavor except life, one can change one's mind and begin anew. In life, by the time the thought occurs, it is too late. Your life is over. I can only hope I have been a loyal husband, a loving father, a faithful friend, because I am out of time to make things right, to make myself better. I talked to Katya today. I begged her to forgive me if my anger has made me cruel. She answered by saying she loves me, that no papa could be better. Her generosity makes me cry.*

These last few months have at least allowed me to plumb the depths of my heart. Every major decision seems suddenly unsound. There is something worse than dying a slow death before you are ready to die. It is to die it with regret.

He asked what was happening in the Waterman case and I told him. He said, *I hope his daughter will visit him before it is too late. I understand why you want to save this man. I hope you succeed.*

■ ■ ■

J effrey called to tell me the successor was ready. I looked it over, made a minor change or two, and said, File it. Then I headed home.

On the way, insulated from the relentlessly positive energy of my indefatigably upbeat associates, I stopped pretending we had a chance. Judges and governors don't care about who you are. All they see is what you did.

I remembered the case of Mario Rodriguez. His life was coming apart. The day he got fired, he went home early and found his wife in bed with another man. Some men throw a highball glass through a window or punch a hole in the wall. Rodriguez fired a gun at his wife's lover and missed, then he shot his wife in the head. His seven-year-old daughter was sleeping in the next room.

When I get appointed to a case, the first thing I do is visualize my clients' crimes. It helps me understand their fury, or their loneliness, or their indifference. For their worst moment, I try to be them. But when I try to be who Rodriguez was that day, Lincoln keeps squeezing into the frame. He is standing at the edge of my visual field, his hands covering his mouth, saying, Dada, stop. And my imagination goes blank.

I understand there is a moral distinction between Rodriguez and a man in free fall who ruins the Baccarat. But there's also a moral distinction between Rodriguez and Ted Bundy. I'm not saying Rodriguez shouldn't have been punished severely. I'm saying he shouldn't have been executed. What good comes from killing such a man? I filed an appeal in his case consisting of a single argument so infirm I have forced myself to forget what it was. I basically just begged the judges to let him live. What he did was punishment enough, I said. He had not hurt anyone during the nine years he'd been in prison, no one except himself. Three times he sliced himself with the handle of a plastic fork he had whittled into a laughable point. Three times they took him to the emergency room, then to a psychiatric unit, then back to death row, where he remained as broken as he was the day he arrived. With two judges dissenting, the court turned me down. I called to tell him. He didn't thank me. His voice was strong. He said, I want you to understand something: I don't care. And he hung up.

■ ■ ■

At home the night of Rodriguez's execution I roasted halibut with sesame, soy, garlic, and wine. I poured Katya a glass of Prosecco and mixed myself a pitcher of Negronis. I made Lincoln a grilled cheese with sliced tomatoes. I carried it to the table and we sat down. Lincoln said, Dada, Nana made me a grill cheese for lunch. Can I have pasta?

I said, I am not a goddamned short-order cook.

Later Katya would tell me that was the moment she concluded I should quit this line of work. She believed I had started showing signs of PTSD. But that evening, she quietly pushed back her chair and walked over to me. She put her hand on my shoulder. She said, I'll fix it.

I covered her hand with mine and stood up. I said, Never mind.

When I returned to the table with the bowl of jumbo shells, Lincoln said, Do what I tell you. I nodded agreement. He said, Close your eyes. I did. He said, Make your mind a blank. Is it blank? I nodded. He said, Good. He took his hands and put them on my face, his palms covering my eyes, his fingers brushing my forehead. He said, In your mind's eye picture you and me and Mama in Park City on a hike. Are you doing that? I nodded. He removed his hands from my face. He said, Okay, you can open your eyes.

He said, Feel better now?

I remembered the day, early in my middle age, when I conceded I would never change the world. I was in New York, on the fifty-first floor looking down. It was dusk. The workers were going home. Thousands and thousands of women and men from everywhere, striding to the bus, to the train, to hail a cab. Tens of thousands of ants, returning to their mounds. That was the moment. We're all just cogs, ants laboring in fields we're too puny to see. All you can change is yourself and your own small corner of this earth. That, and you can help other people change theirs. That's something I've learned.

I said, Yes, yes I do, Linco. Thank you.

He said, You're welcome.

*D*eath is commonly thought to be an occurrence rather than a decision. It isn't, though, and I have made my decision.

I knew. I'd been tired and irritable. The adagio seemed too fast. I knew.

The doctor called this morning. There are at least three new lesions in the brain.

I have ruled out whole-brain radiation therapy. The best it will do is give me four months instead of one, and the price I will pay is lethargy interrupted by vomiting. The surgeon believes the three tumors are accessible (his word), so he wants to cut them out Monday. I told him no thank you. My plan is to die before they have time to do any more damage, and to be the best person I can be until that happens.

The cancer is going to kill me, but I have beaten back the anger. You might consider this a minor achievement, but it isn't, not to me.

I have defeated it entirely. I am no longer angry. I am no longer mad.

■ ■ ■

Dobermans are not natural swimmers. Their short hair does not trap air, and their lean muscle mass creates no buoyancy. In a pool, a Doberman will sink like a stone.

We have a pool. So Katya and I taught Winona to swim and showed her the steps. If she ever fell in, she'd be able to climb out.

But she discovered she liked the water. At first, she would just lie on the steps after a summer run, cooling herself and drinking. Then she began to swim short distances, like a bird testing its wings. A month later she was swimming laps alongside me.

Lincoln liked to throw coins in the water and retrieve them. He would toss in a handful of pennies, put on his mask, and dive to the bottom. When Winona saw this, she panicked. She would leap into the water after him and nosedive down. She would take his arm in her mouth. She was attempting to rescue him.

I could never bring myself to correct this behavior. After several weeks she learned not to worry, but until then, she became so agitated when Lincoln's friends came over to swim, so driven to dive in and attempt a rescue whenever a young boy ducked his head beneath the surface, we had to put her inside and draw the shades so she could not see out to the fun she perceived as danger.

■ ■ ■

The clinic had called. Winona had blood in her feces. She had no appetite. She was constantly listless and intermittently unresponsive. There were sugar and granular casts in her urine, indicating kidney damage from the drugs. Although her earlier blood work had been normal, she now had massively high readings of alanine aminotransferase (ALT) and aspartate aminotransferase (AST), indicating liver damage. A normal range for these enzymes is between 8 and 50 units per liter; Winona's levels had been slightly high on our first trip to the vet. Then they soared to around 7,000. Then they fell back to under 1,000. Now they were near 10,000. I asked the doctor why they were fluctuating so wildly over so short a time span. He said, I am not sure.

I asked, When will you have it under control?

He said, I don't know.

I said, When do you think she can come home?

He said, I don't know that, either.

■   ■   ■

ere's something I've learned: The reason it's easier to be bad than good is that being good takes awareness and effort. You can't just sit there. But all you have to do to be bad is coast.

The Passover Seder is built entirely around the motif that Jews were once slaves. The Haggadah says, Remember you were slaves in the land of Egypt. The institutional memory of subjugation is supposed to foster empathy for today's downtrodden. But if reading one book two nights a year were all it took, we could pass out biographies of Lincoln to every school kid in America and solve all our problems.

Reform Judaism, founded in Europe around the time of the French Revolution, came to America in the mid-nineteenth century. Philip Benjamin helped establish the first Reform synagogue in the United States in Charleston, South Carolina. His son Judah P. Benjamin owned 150 slaves. Jefferson Davis appointed him attorney general of the Confederacy in 1861. Later Davis named him secretary of state.

During the peak of the Civil War, Benjamin lived in Montgomery, Alabama. Of the ten thousand Jewish Confederate soldiers, 130 came from Alabama. I've heard the last Rebel soldier killed in defense of Mobile was a Jewish boy from South Carolina. Did he attend a Seder two days before that city fell to Union forces on April 12, 1865?

A century later the Freedom Riders would arrive in Alabama from the North to help desegregate the South, where they'd be met and violently beaten by members of the KKK on their way home from church. Riding with the blacks into this maelstrom were many Jews. I doubt what differentiated them from the Confederate Jews a century before was keeping kosher or eating matzoh. The difference is the southerners simply coasted.

Two days before Waterman's execution, at shortly after five, the state court ruled against us. The judges didn't bother telling us what was wrong with our argument, or why we'd lost, but one judge did write an illuminating opinion. She said just because we had found a new and clever argument didn't mean we had to raise it.

We'd known this was going to happen. While waiting for the formal announcement, I spent the day writing our appeal to the Supreme Court. I asked Jeffrey and Cara to look it over and file it the next day by noon. I would go to the prison in the morning to tell our client.

At home Katya was sitting upstairs on the sofa in the reading area. There were pages of computer printouts dealing with cancer therapies spilling off her lap, but she wasn't reading. She was holding a mug of tea and staring out the window into the darkness. She said, I am sadder than I thought possible. From the very beginning he told me having the cancer in his brain is the only death he fears. Did he tell you he must have done something to deserve this? I don't know what to say to him.

She looked away from the window and directly at me. Her eyes were puffy and red. She said, What's wrong?

Nothing.

Tell me. What is it?

I said, Don't say anything to him. Just be there for him, and for your mom.

She said, Just being there is not nearly enough.

■ ■ ■

ENDINGS

here we are today and here we are not tomorrow:

if you kick the sand you are likely to raise some dust:

—A. R. AMMONS, "Sphere"

Végre nem butulok torább

(Finally I am becoming stupider no more.)

—Self-written epitaph, PAUL ERDOS

n the first person, beginnings matter more than endings. In the third person, the opposite is true.

And either way, it's best when endings are short, or maybe fast is the better word. Perhaps I am not agnostic on the question I started out with after all. There's greater grief, but in return you get less pain, and much less guilt. If there's no time to think to yourself that it would be better for everyone if the dead man would hurry up and die, you don't have to beat yourself up for having had that thought, like a stomach that growls during an execution because you haven't eaten in two days.

Over the years I have learned guilt is indomitable. But just because you can't subdue it doesn't mean you can't make its agonizing screams a little bit quieter.

■ ■ ■

didn't tell Katya I was going to see him. He was sitting in the rocking chair, facing the lake. He had developed edema and his legs looked like upside-down carrots. He took a blanket draping his shoulders and dropped it across his lap. He said, *The brain surgeon does not return my calls. All I want to ask him is how much longer. If I had to do it over again, I should choose someone who is less skilled as a doctor but more decent as a human being.* I kissed his head. He said, *It's not that I am fearful of death. But the journey is demoralizing and demanding, and my so-called doctors only make it harder.*

He looked at the cover of the book I was holding, Wallace Stevens. He asked, *Will you read?*

Like the first light of evening, as in a room
In which we rest and, for some small reason, think
The world imagined is the ultimate good.

He smiled and closed his eyes and said from memory,

Out of this same light, out of the central mind,
We make a dwelling in the evening air,
In which being there together is enough.

I said, Impressive.

It reminds me of how you say all the time it is better to teach children to be good than not to be bad.

I said, I say it. You did it.

Yes. Irmi and I. I love her so, and my children. If I believed in prayer I would pray they will not miss me so much as I would miss them. His head drooped and I thought he might have fallen asleep. He said, *I hope you are able to save your gangster.*

Me too, but it doesn't look good. He put his hand on mine. I said, You were right. About everything.

He said, *No, I was going to say that. You were right, about everything.*

I said, You play like you practice.

You've got to have chicken to make chicken salad.

I said to him, It ain't over till it's over.

He said, *Touché.*

I walked over to touch him before saying good-bye. His chin had fallen forward again. This time he was sleeping.

It was the last actual conversation we had.

■ ■ ■

W inona was still at the emergency clinic. The vet said she was going to have to spend at least another several nights. I was sitting in our library looking over the Waterman appeal for the Supreme Court when Lincoln got home from school and said he was ready to go visit her. I told him I needed to work for a while. His lower lip started to quiver and his eyes got wet. I said, Go get Mama and we'll go.

Winona was lying on her side, in the middle of the floor in a surgical suite where another vet and two technicians were working on a dog who'd been hit by a car. She had IV tubes running in each front leg and was covered with two quilts and an electric blanket. She raised her head slightly when she saw us but made no move to stand. The memory of the pain in her eyes makes me cry as I sit here, but on that day, with Lincoln there, I held it in. We sat on the floor, the three of us, all stroking her and telling her she'd get better and be home with us soon, even though the vet had pulled me aside as we arrived and told me they still had no idea what was going on. Her blood work continued to show signs of liver failure. She was still bleeding internally, but it was not clear from where. She had not stood since we brought her in days before.

We stayed for over an hour, until her eyes slid shut, and told the vet to call if there were any developments and that no matter what, we'd be back in the morning. Katya asked Lincoln whether he wanted to stop for edamame and vegetable tempura on the way home. He said he wasn't hungry and started to cry. Katya climbed into the backseat and wrapped him in her arms. In the rearview mirror I could see she was crying, too.

Lincoln asked if he could sleep in our room. At three thirty I gave up trying and walked downstairs. I filled a mug with hot water and lemon and carried it outside, but sitting there without Winona I felt bile beginning to rise. I went into the library and sat reading *Falling Water* until the eastern sky turned cobalt and NPR's news came on. Then I went for a run and tried to rehearse the conversation I'd have with Waterman later that day.

On the way to the prison I stopped at the clinic again. Winona seemed even worse than the night before. I curled up in a fetal position, lying on my right side, my nose touching hers, and told her I was sorry. I asked her a question I had just read in the Koethe poem: Why can't the more expansive ecstasies come true? And then I told her they could. I promised if she got better I'd never give her drugs again without doing research first. I promised her I would be a better friend. I said, Your brother and Katya and I need you.

Still she lay there, eyelids shut, with no sign of recognition, and almost no life. I kept talking anyway, hoping my voice was reaching her, clinging to the same baseless faith held by people who swear their brain-dead loved ones can hear. I told her Lincoln loved her. I told her he carried her picture in his pocket and watched it like a television during his meals. I said, He loves you, podjo.

When I said Lincoln's name, Winona opened her eyes and licked my chin.

■ ■ ■

headed due east toward Livingston on Highway 105. At the Lone Star airport, just west of Cut and Shoot, I stopped to watch a pilot do touch-and-go landings in a vintage yellow T-6 Warbird. Peter and I had planned to go fake dogfighting over Lake Conroe in those exact same planes. We never did.

After love, the most potent human emotion is regret. It might be even more potent, because unlike love, you never get past it.

Waterman was already waiting for me. He was eating salad with a plastic fork, spearing pieces of lettuce and cucumber and dunking them into a container of Italian dressing. When he saw me he smiled and wiped his mouth with the back of his sleeve. I said, Who bought you the food?

He said, Chaplain was just here.

I said, I thought you didn't trust that guy. Since when do you do Bible study?

He said, Hey, I'll be dead in two days. Smart white dude in the house next door told me 'bout Pascal's wager. I figure it can't hurt. Anyway, all we really do is talk about how to be a better man.

I said, Who told you?

He said, Nobody told me nothing. But you're here.

He opened a can of iced tea and took a long swallow.

I told him we had lost as expected in the state court and that we were appealing to the Supreme Court. He said, But there's like zero chance they'll rule for me, right?

I said, Pretty close to zero.

He nodded. He said, Worst day I had inside here was when my pop died, and I couldn't be there when they buried him. Didn't even hardly know him, but still. Just a couple of gravediggers throwing dirt on his box.

He leaned forward and held his head in his hands. Without looking up he said, Someone from your office is gonna be there to watch me, right? I waited for him to make eye contact, then I nodded. He said, That's good. Thank you.

One of the things about talking to people whose time of death you could use to set a watch is how aware you become of the emptiness of words. The problem is, unless you play the cello, there isn't any alternative. So I said what I truly felt. I said, I'm really sorry.

He said, I got plans to be buried back home, and I already done gave most of my stuff away, but what's gonna happen with the money I still got in my commissary? They send that to my daughter or what?

How much is it?

Oh, not that much. Maybe seventy-five bucks. Maybe ninety.

I said, I don't know what they do with it. I'll talk to the warden and make sure your daughter gets it.

He nodded. Another thing I've noticed is how people about to die so try to comfort the living. Is it empathy or is it guilt? He said, Relax. Fat lady ain't sung. And he smiled a genuine smile. I returned it with a fake.

I said, I'll see you day after tomorrow.

He said, All right. He touched his hand to the glass, and I touched it back.

I stepped out of the tiny visiting booth and closed the door. Through the window the size of an iPad I watched him take the dressing, drop it on top of the mostly uneaten salad, and push the container away. I banged much harder than necessary on the electric metal door to get the attention of the guard in the control booth. Her head jerked up, her eyes angry, her teeth clenched. Then she saw me, softened, and quickly opened the door.

■　■　■

drove to their house on the lake. Irmi was sitting in the living room reading *Cities of the Plain*. A woman from hospice was packing her bag to leave while her replacement washed her hands in the kitchen sink. I said to Irmi, I think that's the weakest of the three.

She said, I'm enjoying it.

I said, I liked it too. Just not so much as the others. Where are Peter and Katya?

Katya was talking to Peter. With his hospital bed, there was room for only one chair. I was going to ask her how Peter was doing, but I figured I'd wait for Katya to tell me. Ten minutes later she walked in. She kissed me and said, I didn't expect to see you here.

I said, I'm trying to see how many sad conversations I can have in a single day. How is he?

She said, He just stares. I told him it might not be too late to do radiation and shrink the tumors that have grown back. He smiled and squeezed my hand.

I said, Meaning what?

She said, I have no idea. He might not even have understood me.

I said, You think I can go see him?

She said, Sure. He probably won't say anything.

He was lying on a hospital bed. The woman from hospice had

shaved his cheeks. They glistened and smelled like citrus. He turned his head toward the door as I entered and I could see in his eyes he knew me. I'd brought him a volume of Wallace Stevens poems. I held up the copy of *The Palm at the End of the Mind* and said, I'll leave this with Irmi before I leave.

He said, *Über hinaus*—

I touched his ankle. He tried again. He said, *Über hinaus den letzten Gedanken.*

The words came out like he was pouring cold honey. I said, My German is kind of rusty.

He said, *Eiswürfel.*

I'm not sure I understand. Should I get Irmi?

He moved his eyes to the left and said again, *Eiswürfel.*

Next to the bed was a table with a water pitcher. It was full of crushed ice. I poured some into a Styrofoam cup and handed it to him. He said, *Danke.*

I said, Bitte. I'll see you again soon. Don't let Irmi feed you any wild hickory nuts.

I'm pretty sure he was smiling as I walked out. That's how I remember it, anyway. That's how I intend to remember it.

Katya and her mom were sitting next to each other on the sofa. There were two glasses of wine, but neither had drunk a sip. Katya asked me how it had gone. I said, He was talking to me in German. She put her hand on her mother's thigh. I said, Y'all want to go eat dinner?

Irmi said, You two go. I'm tired, and Philip is coming in tonight.

I said, What's Eiswürfel?

Irmi said, It can mean ice cubes.

I said, How about that. I guessed right.

Katya said, I'll see you in the morning, Mama.

Without thinking about it, I drove us to Ninfa's on the east side. It was no longer as hard edged as it had been when Katya and I went there on one of our first dates nine years before. It was Peter's favorite restaurant. He and Irmi would eat an early dinner every two weeks before the theater. The waiter Esteban knew them by name and placed their order when he saw them walking in the door. He was there that night. He asked, How is Señor Peter?

Katya said, Very bad.

Esteban stared at his feet and when he looked back up his eyes were wet. He said, Please tell Señora Irmi I am praying for you. He made a cross on his chest and walked away. Two minutes later he returned with a pitcher of margaritas and a plate of ratones. He said, Con permiso, I will bring you tacos al carbon and mariscos Acapulco. They are Señor Peter's favorites.

Katya's eyes flooded. She said, Thank you, Esteban.

Esteban put his hand on her shoulder. He said, A su servicio.

※ ※ ※

know an artist who sends out invitations to his openings before he's painted a single canvas. I took a clue. When I registered for the marathon I intended to complete for my fiftieth birthday, I paid with a credit card months in advance. I was tied to the mast.

I did my long runs on Fridays. Every Friday morning, after Lincoln left for school, I put on my iPod and plodded around the city for an hour, two hours, three hours, four hours. I'd run through West University, around Rice, through the Village. I'd recite poems I memorized in college and invent Fibonacci sequences. I listened to hundreds of songs. The music did not cause me to enjoy the running.

The injuries came. First my right hamstring then, when it healed, the left. Then my left shin, and my right Achilles tendon after that. I went to Johannes for a massage. He worked on me from the hips down for two solid hours. As I was writing the check he said, Your legs are still a mess.

Two weeks before the race I went on my longest pre-marathon run. When I got home Katya asked me how I felt. I said, I feel like I'm about to throw up.

She said, Yeah. You don't look so good.

I told you: Sometimes you can tell by looking.

That morning there were nearly 30,000 runners. My goal was

not to walk and not to stop, and to finish before they shut down the course. At mile 13 I accepted an orange slice and a glazed donut from two young girls. Someone promised when I hit mile 19, when I turned right on Woodway and spied the buildings on the western edge of downtown rising like a mirage over the Memorial Park's pines, the adrenaline would carry me to the finish. Someone lied.

At mile 21 a hairy fat guy wearing no shirt handed me a beer. You can tell by looking.

You know those tiny reflectors in the middle of the street used to divide the lanes? They stick up maybe a quarter inch above the pavement. At mile 11, I tripped on one and nearly fell. At mile 16 I stumbled on another. At mile 22, when I tripped for the third time, a young woman wearing pink and looking like she had run maybe a mile said to me, You know, you really should pick up your feet when you run. I interpreted that as flirting.

At the finish line there was a volunteer holding one banana. Of all the people she saw, she gave that banana to me. She could tell by looking, too.

At home I spent an hour in the hot tub, thirty minutes in the steam, then thirty more in the hot tub. I showered and got in bed. Lincoln served me another banana and an orange. For dinner I feasted on two buffalo burgers and drank two beers. I fell asleep in the massage chair and had a dream. I dreamed the person who draped the finisher's medal around my neck was Waterman. He was smiling like a proud papa. He said, I knew you could do it.

■ ■ ■

Peter used to tell me the ordinary mortal can know only two things with certainty. One is the difference between right and wrong, the other is love. Katya and I drove to the lake to have a drink with her mom. Irmi poured two glasses of white wine and handed me a lowball glass and a bottle of Woodford Reserve. We sat in the living room and watched the ducks prowl for a meal. Katya and I had broken ground on a new house we were building. Irmi asked about the progress. She asked about Waterman. She asked if we were hungry.

Peter was lying behind us, on a bed with rolling wheels supplied by hospice. His eyes were open but fixed. He was wearing a hospital gown and an adult diaper. He was not speaking a word.

When he had decided to have no more surgery, he told me, *There is an advantage to knowing you are going to die. I do not mean in the abstract way we all know we are mortal. I mean knowing more or less exactly when you will expire so you can circle the date on your calendar and not leave tasks undone. Your clients and I are who I mean. People in a plane crash know, but not with enough time to reflect or to plan.*

He had taken the money he had saved to play and moved it into a trust for Irmi and his kids. He'd sold his sailboat and organized his garage. He finished the book he was reading and cleaned out his desk. Watching him strip down his life, I became the opposite of a hoarder. Behind Katya's and Lincoln's backs, I secretly throw things away.

Irmi opened her nostrils wide, like a bird dog on the scent. She said, Will you please help me? I followed her to where Peter was lying on his back. She asked me to lift his hips, and when I did she removed his soiled diaper, cleaned him, and put on another. She lifted the blanket to his shoulders and kissed his forehead. I looked into his flat eyes and said, You do not need to worry about your family.

I think if he heard me, he didn't understand.

■ ■ ■

Waterman was thirty-two hours away from death. It was 10 A.M. Tuesday, the day before his scheduled lethal injection. The guard at the gate asked me who I was there to see. When I told him he waved me in, not bothering with the normal routine of looking in my trunk, glove box, and engine block. He said, If I am here when you come out, just wave. If there's someone else, you're number twelve on the list.

I parked far from the gate. I needed the walk. I was still in the car, making sure to leave behind all the items prison rules forbid—cell phones, paper money, sunglasses, newspapers, hats—when I got a text from a number I did not recognize. It said, It is urgent that I talk to you. It is about your case. I remembered the note I found on my car weeks before. It was still right there, folded neatly in my back pocket, exactly where I had forgotten it. The number was the same. I wrote a note to myself, reminding me to reply, and left it on the dashboard.

Waterman was in the cage waiting for me. He was eating a Twix bar and drinking a soda. I said, Unusual choice.

He did not smile. He said, I usually treat myself on Friday. Don't think I'll be havin' another Friday. I asked whether he planned to do his thousand push-ups in the morning. He said, Probably so. Plan on making my last day a good one.

I told Waterman I would try to think of something else to file, but

I didn't think I'd come up with anything. I told him I would write a letter to the governor, but the governor never intervened. In fact, he sometimes did not even reply to my requests. I continued to ask just because I couldn't bear not to. Waterman said, That's all right, Professor. If it's time it's time.

We talked about the cases of some of the guys he was friends with on the row. He asked how Cara and Jeffrey were holding up after Starret. We talked a lot about his daughter. He asked me whether the victim's relative was still alive and whether he would be a witness. When I told him I wasn't sure, he asked whether, if the man was there, it would be all right to tell him to his face he was sorry. He asked after the students who'd been in the county jail. We talked about what the routine would be like the following day. He asked whether the execution would be painful, and even though I don't have a clue, I told him no.

We sat there until the visitors were gone and the transport teams had taken all the inmates back to the row. We sat there while Sergeant Scott finished her paperwork and checked it twice. We sat there even after she asked me four times to wrap it up then went and stacked fifty plastic chairs upside down on the Formica ledge.

We sat there until Eddie finally said, I better get on back to the block 'fore I get one of these brothers in trouble. His forced smile didn't mask his fear. He squatted down, back against the door, with his arms behind him so the guard could reach through a slot and cuff his wrists. When they opened the door, one of the three guards said something to him I couldn't hear, and Waterman tried to laugh, but he couldn't. He looked back over his shoulder at me and said, Relax, and please don't be beatin' yourself up. I'll be talking to you again tomorrow. Then he walked away.

I watched him go, watched him turn the corner, watched him head off to bed for the final time. I stood but then sat, not yet able to leave. I stared at the empty hall, thinking maybe he'd come back, thinking maybe he'd ask the guards to bring him back. They would have done it, I think. He still had half his candy bar left to go. It was lying right there on the graffiti-covered shelf, untouched in its shiny foil sleeve.

I do not know how many minutes passed. I heard gates clanging shut and corrections officers laughing as they headed to their trucks. On the control booth glass I saw a reflection of green numbers blinking on a computer screen that had been obsolete for twenty years. I sat watching the sky turn gray through a window the inmates couldn't see. Sergeant Scott walked over again. She put her hand on my shoulder and said, They're coming in to mop the floors. You want to stay a little longer? I shook my head and followed her through the electric door.

■ ■ ■

called the number the text had been sent from. I got a generic voice mail message. I left my name, my office phone, and the number I was calling from, even though whomever I was calling had it already. When I got to the office two hours later Cara said, Someone called and said he had information about why the guards wouldn't talk to us.

I said, Yeah, I got a text. Who was it? Did he leave a number?

She said, He said you were the only person he'll talk to. He said he'd call back.

I went to the conference room and lay down on the floor in another futile effort to unknot my back. Five minutes later Cara and Jeffrey came in. He tossed me my Super Ball and said, If the guy calls back, maybe he'll have something to say we can use for a successor. I sat up and for the next hour the three of us brainstormed how to construct a legal claim on top of a fact we didn't know. To build an argument we made up the fact, made it into the perfect fact, the only fact we could think of how to use. We decided someone had muzzled the guards.

Finally I said, This is a waste of time. We don't even know the story. And frankly, even if it turns out to be the greatest story ever written, it won't get us a stay. It might get us disbarred, but it won't get a stay. I don't want to start yanking Waterman's chain. He's ready. We file something else, he'll just have to pace around that holding cell three extra hours before they kill him. Pull the damn plug.

I poured three fingers of barrel proof Willet into a highball glass and held up the bottle. They both shook their heads. Cara was clenching her teeth and I thought Jeffrey might cry. I said, Fuck it. Y'all want to tinker all night, be my guest. If the guy calls back, tell him to call my cell.

Katya and Lincoln were sitting at the kitchen table. She was helping him study for his test on the Middle Ages while I fixed pasta and a salad. I said, Are you two gaslighting me? What does that question have to do with the exam?

Katya had asked Lincoln why the man's daughter ran away. Lincoln had answered that she was upset because her father cut off people's heads.

Lincoln said, Dada, in case you forgot, the book we read is *The Executioner's Daughter.*

I said, Yeah, but I didn't think it was actually about an executioner.

He said, With that title, what did you think it would be about?

In the middle of dinner I got a text. It said, Meet me at the House of Pies. I have what you need.

It was nine o'clock. I told Lincoln good night and Katya not to wait up, and I got in my car.

At the diner the dinner crowd was mostly gone and the insomniacs were yet to come. One booth had a gay couple and two others had parents with their kids. There was a white guy so covered with tattoos he looked black sitting at the counter next to an Asian girl with three rings piercing her lower lip. They were sharing a piece of coconut cream pie, and against my will I found myself thinking they looked sweet.

Sitting alone in a booth near the back was a middle-age man wearing tan Sansabelt trousers and a double-knit green shirt. He had Vitalis-slicked hair and was watching the door with an untouched mug of coffee. He had to be my man. I introduced myself. He said, Get away from me you pervert before I call the cops.

I said, Sorry pal, mistaken identity. I took a stool three down from the young lovers and whirled around 180 degrees to watch the door. I checked my phone every five minutes. At midnight I bought a Bavarian chocolate pie so the night would not be a complete bust and headed home.

Katya had fallen asleep with the TV on. The chefs on *Chopped* were making a dessert featuring smoked oysters. If there was any symbolism God was expecting me to perceive, she overestimated me. I kissed Katya, checked on Lincoln, and went into my study. I called the office. I was hoping for voice mail but prepared for the worst. Sure enough, Jeffrey answered. I said, What the fuck are you doing?

He said, I came up with a 1983 claim. I'm almost through writing it up.

A 1983 claim is a civil rights lawsuit. In a phrase, someone who files this kind of suit is accusing the state of not playing by the rules. We had used the technique in numerous cases to challenge the legality of the chemical cocktail used to carry out executions. Although many other lawyers were still pursuing those challenges, I had concluded they were just a sport that had no prospect of helping my clients, so I had abandoned them. I said, I could hardly be more skeptical, but I'll read it. I'll be in around six.

The essence of Jeffrey's argument was that Waterman had a right to request clemency. When the state interfered with our efforts to interview guards as part of our clemency effort, the state had violated Waterman's rights. I said, Jeffrey, it's brilliant.

And it was. Then I said, But we can't file it.

He stared at me, crestfallen. I said, In the first place, we have no idea whether anyone interfered with anybody. In the second place, even if someone did, we have no idea whether it was someone who works for the government. In the third place, even if someone did, and even if it was Governor Perry himself, the Board of Pardons and Paroles is made up of a bunch of people who don't even believe in clemency. It wouldn't matter if every last guard in the joint wanted Waterman to live. So where's the harm? I don't even know why we bother with these things.

I waited for him to argue. He looked past me, out my window, at the vacant lot across the street littered with stained mattresses and broken beer bottles. He said, I agree. I just couldn't sleep. It made me feel better to write it.

I said, Why don't you go home and try. All we're going to do today is twiddle our thumbs for the next twelve hours.

He said, I'll take a short nap in my office. He picked up the pages from the corner of my desk and dropped them in the shredder. I watched him climb the stairs to his couch. He's twenty-nine years old and puts in 150 miles a week on his bike. He was clutching the banister like an old man.

■ ■ ■

never think about being dead in twelve hours. I think about being dead tomorrow. Having to pass through a period where I'd ordinarily be asleep stymies me. Did Waterman go to bed last night?

My eyes were burning but I knew I wouldn't sleep. I downloaded a Regina Spektor record and listened while I played a few hands of poker. I checked the price of airfares to Vegas. I went to Amazon and bought *On Beauty* by Zadie Smith and then tried to read a paper about Shizuo Kakutani's fixed-point theorem. I didn't understand most of it, but I kept reading anyway. Awareness of my limitations used to depress me. Now it's the foundation of everything I know.

Cara walked in at eight with a box of donuts and a gallon of coffee. I was in my office, swinging a baseball bat at a punching bag. She stood in the doorway and said, Where's Jeffrey? His car's here.

I said, Dreaming.

She stared at me and said, I swear you need a translator. Did the mystery man call you back?

I said, Yep. He stood me up. I won't be asking him out again. Let's talk about getting DNA testing for Anthony.

Our next client facing death, Broderick Anthony, was scheduled to die in three weeks. We had found some frozen hairs, recovered from the hand of the murder victim, that had never been tested. We wanted to get them analyzed. If there was root material on the hair strands, we might be able to get a genetic profile, and maybe that profile would be in a law enforcement database, and if it was, we might be able to prove our client's persistent claim of innocence.

She said, Now?

I said, I've got a couple of hours before I have to drive to Huntsville. She shook her head, dropped her jacket on the floor, pulled a laptop out of her bag, and sat down at my conference table.

Two hours later, as Cara and I were finishing the Anthony road map, Jeffrey walked in. He said, I think we're going to get a stay.

I said, I know you think that. You amuse me. Every execution around here is Groundhog Day. I'm going to Huntsville. Call me when we get denied.

Jeffrey said, *If* we get denied.

I said, Yeah. That's what I meant.

To Cara, who would be witnessing the execution, I said, I'm not going to wait around for time of death. I'll see you back in Houston tonight.

As I arrived at the Hospitality House in Huntsville I got another text. It said, I apologize for last night. Something came up. Please call me.

I deleted the text and walked inside. Two of Waterman's pen pals were there. Valerie had arrived from France three days earlier. Guri, from Norway, had been living in a Huntsville motel for a week. She and Waterman talked about getting married. Both women were sitting in vinyl-covered recliners, leaning forward, holding mugs of tea in their hands, portrait models of grief. Two years earlier Valerie had asked me to please keep her informed about our plans for the case. I said, Our plans are confidential. You can know what we've done after we do it.

Katya tells me I have issues with trust. She might be right. But I don't know these people. They're halfway around the world sitting in cafés, reading about how terrible America is. They could enlist in a thousand different causes. They could befriend five billion people. But they seek out killers in Texas. I admire their dedication, but what possible reason could I have to trust them?

Maybe, Katya says, because it's people like them who change the world.

Guri walked over and hugged me. Valerie did not stand up. She said, Is there news?

I said we would not hear from the Supreme Court until less than an hour before the execution. She asked why they take so long. I said, Because this is a game to them. Because they are assholes. Because they pretend like there is not a human life at stake while they claim there is nothing they can do.

She said, Like the Germans.

I said, No. It's not the Holocaust. That's a ridiculous analogy.

One thing I've learned about extremist views is they are attractive because they are simple. But ethics is the one domain where Occam's razor is wrong. Even people who disagree about something basic and fundamental still agree much more frequently than they don't. Judge Norton, the court of appeals judge so eager to see Waterman dead, was contemptible, but he probably loves his son as much as I love mine.

Valerie looked at me like she'd been slapped, or maybe betrayed. I said, There's a difference between doing something bad and allowing something bad to happen. I agree with you that they're both bad, but they're not the same.

She said, Except to the victim.

She had me there. I said, The Supreme Court waits until the last possible minute so we do not have time to do anything else. The last thing they ask me when they call to tell me we've lost is whether I plan to pursue any more options. I think I might start saying yes, just to ruin their day.

Valerie and Guri smiled. I told them I was going to the prison, that if there was good news, I would call them, but that if I had not called or returned by five thirty, they should assume the worst. Guri walked over and sat on the arm of Valerie's chair. She draped her arm over Valerie's shoulders. I nodded to them, turned up my collar, and stepped outside. Three blocks away, my client was in a holding cell, eight steps away from the room where he'd be dead in two more hours.

Most prisons are in the middle of nowhere. Not this one. The Walls Unit sits smack-dab in downtown Huntsville, right there on 12th Street, surrounded by diners and tree-lined residential streets. I desperately wanted the Supreme Court to call before I saw him. I wanted to be able to tell him in person we had lost, rather than have to call him after I'd gone. I stalled by walking right past the prison to the Farmhouse Café. It was packed. Executions in Huntsville are so common the locals don't even know they're occurring. A waitress called me *hon* and led me to a Formica-covered deco table that was not a reproduction. I asked her for a slice of chocolate pie and a bottomless cup of coffee. She said, That's my favorite. Back in a sec. I drank one swallow and the phone rang. It was Jeffrey.

I said, Yeah?

He said, No news. I just wanted to get you before you went inside. Cara's on her way up.

I said, Okay. Thanks. I'm just sitting here teaching a master class in avoidance behavior. I'm going inside now.

I put a five-dollar bill on the table and called the warden's secretary and told her I would be there in three minutes. She was at the door waiting for me. I passed through two electronic doors, crossed a courtyard, walked through another door, and there was Waterman, sitting on a bare mattress, writing in a spiral notebook. He looked up, and he really did look serene, like a man whose parachute has just opened, slowing his plummet, and bathing him in quiet.

Three guards stepped to the end of the corridor, as far away from us as they could get. He said, I was just writing you a letter.

I said, The Supreme Court just called. We lost.

He said, Oh. Well, that's okay. I knew we were going to lose. I been sayin' all my good-byes. You don't need to be worryin' 'bout me. I'm prepared. I really am.

I said, Why are you writing me a letter? I told you I'd see you.

He said, Yeah, I know. But writing's easier for me than saying things out loud. I can hand it to you when I'm done if you don't want to be gettin' mail from me after I'm dead.

I said, However you want to play it is okay with me. I looked to my left. One of the guards who'd been listening to us dropped his head. Waterman gave me messages to deliver: He asked me to tell his mother he loved her. He wanted me to tell his daughter he wished he had been there for her. He told me how grateful he was to the lawyers and guards who had tried to help him.

He said, Ain't you gonna write it down?

I said, I promise you I'll remember every word.

Then we were quiet. The same guard made eye contact with me and looked toward the door. I shook my head. He mouthed, Okay.

Waterman said, Only reason I wanted to go to my dad's funeral was so I could tell him it wasn't his fault. I was the one who made the bad choices. That's all I wanted to say to him.

I said, If you forgave him, he knows.

He said, Ain't a matter of forgiving. Wasn't nothing to forgive.

I said, What about your mom?

He looked past me, through the small window in the dungeon door. It was dusk. He said, I did what I did, not her.

I had nothing to say, so I said nothing. I needed to leave, and I had to stay. I stood there for ten minutes more, until the warden walked in and told me it was almost time for me to go. I touched both my palms to the mesh between us. Waterman walked over and touched his to mine. He held them there, and so did I. I said, I've never wanted to win for someone more than I wanted to win for you. I'm sorry.

He said, Hey, man, I know all that. And he smiled, a real smile. He said, Professor, you been there with me the whole way, every step and then some. Thank you. I mean that. Thank you.

And he called me by my name.

I said, I'll see you down the road. And I walked out before I could start to cry.

Back at the hospitality house Valerie and Guri were sitting on the porch smoking. As I walked up the phone rang. It was Jeffrey calling to tell me we had lost. He said, Two dissents.

I reported the news to the two women. Guri said, Do you have to call Eddie now?

I said, I already told him.

She said, What? When?

Valerie said, Before you knew? What if you had been wrong?

I said, I wasn't wrong.

■ ■ ■

hree reporters and Cara watched Waterman die. Miss Mc-
Clain's only living relative was not there. He told a reporter
from the local paper he had no desire for the state to kill someone on his behalf. He said his aunt would not have wanted it, either.
The reporter asked him whether he had heard about Waterman's
supposed transformation in prison. He replied, Miss, if that is true I
am pleased to learn it, but I must confess that the murderer's biography is not something that interests me. I have been busy living my
own life, not paying attention to someone else's, or wishing for someone else's to end.

The reporter played the tape for me and asked if I had a comment, I said no and thought to myself, I'd like to know that man.

Guards from the tie-down team strapped Waterman to the gurney
at exactly 6 P.M. A technician inserted IV lines that would carry three
drugs. First a barbiturate to sedate him, followed by a paralytic agent
so the witnesses would not see him convulse, and finally a drug to
induce cardiac arrest. When the curtain separating the execution
chamber from the witness room opened, his right leg was bouncing
up and down. His final statement was short. Waterman turned his
head toward Cara and thanked his lawyers. Then he looked up at the
ceiling and swallowed. He apologized again for all his mistakes, in-

cluding, as he put it, the granddaddy of a mistake that got him there, and he said the responsibility was only his. He told his mom he loved her. He told his daughter he wished he had been there for her. He thanked the prison staff for their professionalism and courtesy, and then he said, Warden, I am ready. He was dead at 6:19.

As I was driving home my phone rang. It was Sharice. She said, Mr. Dow, I was listening to the prison show on the Internet and they said the Supreme Court turned my daddy down. Is that true?

I said, Yes it is. I'm sorry. Your father is dead.

The whir of my tires on the highway almost covered up the sound of her tears. I heard only the barest sniffle. She asked whether there would be a funeral, and I told her where it would be. She said, I want to see him before they close the casket and give him a letter I wrote. Can I do that? I told her she could. She said, I just wanted to tell him I forgive him, and that I love him. I wrote it last year and I never did send it. I meant to mail it, and I never did.

Then I heard a sob. She hung up without saying good-bye.

■ ■ ■

study the faces of the dead. Dead faces have no attitudes. They don't try to fool you by pretending to be innocent or tough, or by pretending to understand what is coming, or not to. Here's something I've learned: Sometimes you don't really know someone until you've seen him dead.

By the time my clients die, I've known them for an average of six-point-eight years. I know their names, where they were born, and where they went to school. I know their grades, the number of days they were absent, and when they dropped out. I know the jobs they held, the drugs they used, and the crimes they committed, including the ones they got away with. I've read their medical records and reports of prior incarcerations. I've met their siblings and their parents and sometimes their children. I've talked to almost every person they've ever known. I know the names of the people they abused, and who abused them, and I could recite for you like multiplication tables the details of that abuse. I know whether they are smart or average or dumb, or whether they just pretend to be. I know what they are good at and what they're scared of and whether they like to read. I know how much they sleep, how often they masturbate, and what junk food they like to eat. I know every single thing about them, and I still don't know them at all—not until I see their faces for the first time without a mask, once they're dead, and no longer hiding from me. The fifty muscles that shape the face soften like lard and reveal more truth than open eyes.

Cara had arranged to recover the body. She was going to the funeral later that day. Not me. I'm a heathen. I wanted to visit without the tribalism and superstition that fills the air like humidity in what believers call houses of God. I drove to the funeral home. A man whose face was puttied with pancake makeup escorted me in silence to a room with a window unit air conditioner dripping water onto the rotting sill. He nodded and left, and it was just me and an open casket.

Eddie was smiling. His lips were deep purple, like a ripe black plum. That seemed strange to me, because they'd been pink as bubble gum twenty-one hours ago, which is how long had passed since I'd seen him alive.

I'd driven back to Houston and bought the team who'd worked on his case three rounds of drinks at Warren's. Cara said, When I walked out after the execution a reporter asked me whether I could go back in and come out again, wiping tears from my eyes. He wanted to get it on camera.

Jeffrey had already heard this story and was studying his beer. I said, What did you say?

Cara said, I told him sure, and I walked back inside. I left through a side door. I hope he's still standing there.

I lifted my glass. I said, To small victories.

I walked across the street to Frank's and ordered a pizza for Lincoln and me and a plate of pasta for my wife. I drank a bottle of St. Arnold's while I waited and read through my email. There was a message from the date who had jilted me. He (or she) apologized again and begged to see me. I shook my head and watched the Hispanic kid ladle sauce onto our pie. I said, Querría mucha salsa, por favor.

He said, Sí, señor, and ladled on another scoop.

Katya was waiting for me in the kitchen when I walked in the door. She knows the difference between the ones I can shake off and the ones that bother me a lot. She hugged me, and we stood there. She's learned about silence, too. Lincoln came in from the library. He said, Oh, goodie. It's Frank's. Thanks for letting me stay up late.

I said, You're welcome. But it was Mama's idea. Don't forget to thank her.

He said, I already did that.

I got another text from the mystery person. It said, I will be at the House of Pies in one hour. Please come. Katya asked me what it was, and I told her it was nothing.

Lincoln said, Hey Dada, how long until you're not so glum?

I said, By the time you carry this pizza and a beer into the library, amigo.

He said, Yay.

Katya and I followed him, holding hands.

My clients and their families aren't the only ones I know. Sometimes I also know the loved ones left behind by murder. I might see them in the courtroom or on the TV news. I might read about them in the paper. Some have sent me emails. A few have even called. But the most important thing about them is what it feels like to be them, and that is something I don't ever want to know.

While we ate I got three more texts. The first said, Are you here? I muted my phone and deleted them as they arrived. There are two kinds of people in the world: people who do the right thing, and people who don't. Doing the right thing too late puts you in the latter group.

After Katya and I put Lincoln to bed, I told her the story. She said, Aren't you going to respond to the person?

I said, Nope.

She didn't push me. Katya conserves her moral leverage for things that matter.

I fell asleep reading a biography of John Brown. After my dad, he was my first hero. In ninth grade I memorized his closing statement to the twelve men who sent him to hang. *I have, may it please the court, a few words to say.* He wasn't a suicide bomber. He was willing to die, but he didn't want to. He said, *Now, if it is deemed necessary that I should forfeit my life for the furtherance of the ends of justice, and mingle my blood further with the blood of my children, and with the blood of millions in this slave country whose rights are disregarded by wicked, cruel, and unjust enactments, I say: let it be done.* I don't know how you deliberately execute a bad person, much less a good one. I like to think Brown believed being a better person made him a better dad. The last thing he told his children was to be good haters.

If you can identify the right people to hate, that's pretty good advice.

■ ■ ■

B ut what I had told Lincoln earlier was a lie. When you can save someone's life by pulling certain levers, and the person dies, it means you've pulled the wrong ones. Saying there's plenty of blame to spread around is an empty bromide that privileges self-preservation and deception over truth. But I wasn't going to let myself be deceived, so I pulled a lemon from our tree and squeezed it into a mug of boiling water and carried it outside.

I missed the dog. I heard frogs croaking nearby and in the distance a train, and with everyone I love asleep, I felt all alone. I watched the tree and waited for Waterman to appear and absolve me my error, but he did not. No one else did, either. I remembered a couplet from Ammons: *I do the ones I love no good: / I hold their pain in my hands and toss it in the moonlight.* I looked again to the empty tree. Above me a heavy fog was hiding the waning crescent moon.

I went to the garage to retrieve the letter Waterman handed me ten hours before. I had placed it inside a slim volume of Ammons I keep in my car. Surely it was happenstance Waterman's letter book-marked verse 143, where Ammons said: *by the time you amount to something / the people you meant it to mean something to are dead and you / are left standing there, your honors in your hands.* Waterman had written, *Thank you for being my friend.*

A year ago I woke with a vise gripping my chest. My fingers tingled and I was too dizzy to stand. I said to Katya, I think we need to go to the emergency room. Six hours of testing later, the ER doctor told me I did not have a heart attack. I did not have an embolism or an aortic dissection. I had pericarditis brought on by a virus. I could go home.

But you can be looking for one thing and find another. The doctor discovered my blood pressure medicine was not working, and my pressure was dangerously high. He sent me to a specialist who spent six months trying combinations of six drugs, and nothing seemed to work. I remembered something Peter had told me. He'd said, *Only nonscientists think trial and error is not true science.* Maybe, but all their trials were error. I said to my doctor, You think I should try less stressful work?

The doctor replied, That might not be a bad idea.

When I reported the conversation to Katya and Lincoln, Lincoln said, I don't know, Dada. I think you need to keep trying to help people.

I said, What do you mean by *need*, amigo?

He said, What do you mean?

Lincoln has an iPhone app that plays high-frequency tones he can hear but I cannot. Kids see truths that to adults with inflated egos and hyper–self-awareness—adults like me—remain obscure. I said, I get it Linco. Never mind.

■ ■ ■

have happily married friends who love their spouses and kids, but can't wait to spend a night at home alone. But they don't have my job. When Katya and Lincoln are away, all I can think about are my clients' victims, and the loved ones they left behind. I sit outside with a bourbon or a beer and imagine all the ways they or I might die. In my mind I write a revision of *Harold and Maude*, only in my version, prolific death is untempered by sardonicity or wit.

I've infected Katya, too. The first night Lincoln spent away from us, we sat in the library with the TV on mute until our pasta got cold and I fell asleep balancing an untouched drink on my chest. The next day we got to the school an hour early to greet the bus bringing him home.

I don't know if I've learned anything more important than to leave nothing unsaid.

I left a note on my pillow telling Katya where I was and I drove to the vet. It was nearly 3 A.M. Yellowing fluorescent bulbs buzzed like mosquitoes in the empty room. The technician sitting at the desk didn't seem surprised to see me.

I said, Good evening, or maybe it's good morning. I tried to smile, and she walked me back to Winona's cage.

My dog's eyes were closed. When I placed my hand on her head she didn't stir. I said, No matter how much I've taught you, podjo, you've taught me more.

She did not respond to my voice. I said, You've made me a better person, Winona, and Lincoln says you've made me a better dad.

This time when I said Lincoln's name, she didn't open her eyes.

I touched her face. Her breath was slow and her gums were the color of chalk. I leaned down to kiss her snout, and I felt her whiskers tickle my chin. I rubbed the inside of her ear with the pad of my thumb.

I sat there, and I cried. I said, I love you, podjo.

■ ■ ■

When Katya and I got to the lake the woman from hospice was on her way out. She reminded me of Sergeant Scott from death row, and I stared at her until Katya clasped my elbow and said, Are you okay?

Peter was lying there in the living room, motionless and silent. The woman from hospice had turned him onto his left side because his right buttock had a bedsore oozing pus. Katya picked up his hand and said something to him. He did not respond. I put my hand on Katya's head but said nothing to her dad. Irmi wanted me to take Peter's kayaking gear. I did not need it, but I didn't say no.

We stopped at El Tiempo on the way home. Through dinner I held Katya's forearm like a raft. I think I drank a pitcher of margaritas. I do not remember what I ate. Katya drove us home and must have carried me upstairs. The phone rang at two. Peter was dead.

We got to the lake two hours before dawn. Peter was in the same place we'd seen him a few hours before, still on the hospital bed, his feet pointed toward the water. Irmi was sitting next to him, holding his hand. A year before he was muscular and lean. He'd go out in the morning for a short hike and be gone until sunset. Dead he weighed ninety-eight pounds. I studied his face, too. I wondered whether Irmi had closed his eyes. He did not look serene. He was sixty years old.

I sat between Irmi and Katya at the kitchen table and wrote the obituary by hand on a yellow legal pad while Irmi kept stroking Peter's face. If everybody on earth was loved by someone as much as Peter was loved by her, there would be neither warfare nor hate. I believe that.

Irmi asked me to call the funeral home. The mortician wanted to come recover the body right away. Irmi told me to tell him not yet. They could come in the afternoon. She was not ready for him to be gone.

This, in a nutshell, is the difference between my wife's family and me. To me, he'd been gone already for days.

We stayed with Irmi that night, her first as a widow. The next morning at dawn I was making coffee when the sun punched a hole through the thick stratus clouds and birds came pouring through. Fish thrashed near the surface of the lake. Deer came to graze in the yard. It is possible there are natural explanations for all these phenomena, but I am going to believe they were Peter, coming to say good-bye.

At the funeral a family friend played Bach on an acoustic guitar. Peter's colleagues talked about what a formidable scientist he was. They described his innovative work involving detergents in language I couldn't understand. The women and men who worked for him remembered his decency and goodness in words that I could.

I recounted his last six months for the people there who didn't know, and then I read a Wallace Stevens poem. I was reading it for him, and I am positive I felt him smile. I told his friends something he said to me I thought they might like to hear. He had said, *I used to wonder which would be worse: to live forever, or never to have lived at all.* He was holding a picture of Irmi, Katya, and Phil. He looked at it and pressed it to his chest. He said, *That is one question to which I am certain I have learned the answer.*

■ ■ ■

incoln asked Katya to tell him the story about the hickory nuts. She and her dad had been hiking outside Durango. He was a one-man outdoor school. He wiped his hands on an aspen and told her its bark had salicylic acid, a natural sunscreen. He pointed out edible flowers. He taught her the names of a dozen different plants. *And these,* he said, picking several from a tree, *are wild hickory nuts.* He held some out to her but she waved them off. She ate her peanut butter sandwich instead. Peter said, *Suit yourself,* and he ate them all.

A quarter mile down the trail, he threw up for the first time. Two hundred yards farther, he threw up again. Lincoln said, After he realized they weren't hickory nuts did he learn to be more careful?

Katya said, Not exactly. He told me sometimes you have to make a mistake so you won't make it again.

Lincoln said, That's what Dada says.

Katya said, Yes, but Dada keeps making them over and over.

Lincoln laughed and said, That's true. He looked at me standing there, pretending to be hurt. He said, Well, Dada, it is.

Lincoln stopped being purely happy when he discovered mystery. We were in Utah. Katya was dancing at a competition in Manhattan. I was sitting in the living room, eating my dinner and reading Elizabeth McCracken's memoir about the only tragedy I think I couldn't survive: losing a child. Lincoln sent me a text. It read, I'm sad and I can't sleep. I texted him back, Come down here with me. He carried his pillow into the living room. He lay down on the sofa. I put my hand on his head until he pushed it away.

Earlier that afternoon, we had been hiking with the dog. He was explaining to me how he visualized the workings of his brain. He said, There are lots of little people, I call them Lincoln-people, and they are trying to figure out why I'm sad. But the secret is locked in a safe, and they can't figure out how to open it.

I said, That reminds me of René Descartes, Linco. He was a philosopher who lived more than 350 years ago. He had this idea that the body and soul are different. If I chop off your arm, you'd still be Lincoln, but if you changed the way you think, you'd be a different person.

He said, I get it.

I said, Am I boring you, amigo?

He said, No, I think it's interesting.

It was early July. I had been letting him stay up late, but no matter what time he goes to bed, he is up at six. The night before, when he told me he was sad, I said, It's because you're tired, amigo.

He said, No, I'm tired because I can't sleep, and I can't sleep because I'm sad.

Yes, but you're sad because you're tired.

He said, It is not a chicken-or-egg problem, Dada. I was sad first.

We were three weeks away from his eighth birthday. I said, Then we need to figure out why you're sad.

He said, It started at the end of school.

I said, Did something happen at school that you didn't tell me or Mama about?

No.

Did you see something that upset you?

No.

Katya called. Lincoln answered and put her on speaker. She had won first place in her division. Normally Lincoln would have sung and danced, but all he said was Congratulations, Mama. After we hung up Lincoln said, I don't understand why I'm alive. What is life, anyway?

I said, Amigo, there are some questions no one knows the answers to.

He said, That makes me sad.

I remembered that exchange on the way to the veterinary clinic. The night before I called my cousin Benjamin. He's an oncologist. He knows everything about blood. He is the one who told me if it was a human it would be liver failure. I said, Can a liver fail, recover, fail, recover, and fail again, all in a matter of hours?

He said, Liver function labs can certainly fluctuate significantly.

261

But as far as a liver failing and recovering repeatedly over that time period, I've never heard of it.

Winona's personal vet sent us to the specialist because she was stymied. Now the specialist was stymied, too. He led us into a room where Winona was lying on a quilt, shrugged his shoulders, and left us there. Lincoln lay down on his belly, his nose touching the dog's. Katya and I sat cross-legged on either side of him, one hand on our son, the other on our dog. Winona's eyes were open but still. Her breathing was so shallow her rib cage barely raised. A technician opened the door to see whether we had gone. I said, Is there a time limit or something? She said there wasn't. I told her I'd let them know when we were leaving.

We sat that way for more than an hour, until Winona was asleep and the sky was dark, and we heard dinging from the microwave as the skeleton crew began to heat their evening meals. Walking to the car Lincoln said, It's dinnertime but I'm not very hungry. I think I'm going to go straight to bed. Tomorrow during art I'm going to make Winona a get well card. Can we take it to her when I get home from school?

I told him we could.

■ ■ ■

What is an acceptable margin of error when you are deciding whether to end a life? I used to be in favor of assisted suicide, but now I'm not so sure. You can care too little, or you can care too much, and either way, someone dies who shouldn't.

Five minutes after Lincoln left for school the clinic called. The doctor told me Winona had gotten significantly worse overnight. She was listless and unresponsive. She had lost bladder control. I asked him whether it was time. He said, I think so.

She was lying on her right side on a pallet of quilts, covered by heavy blankets. Katya sat cross-legged in front of her, caressing Winona's snout with her right hand and rubbing her ear with her left. Winona did not acknowledge her touch. I was pacing back and forth, paralyzed. They had already shaved her left front leg. The doctor walked in and kneeled before her. When he tried to insert the IV needle, Winona raised her head, drew her leg back, and batted him away. Katya said, She's not ready. The doctor looked at her, then at me, and when I said nothing, he walked out.

Winona was still again. Her belly was so full of fluid it looked like she'd swallowed a basketball. When I touched it, I heard liquid sloshing around like a flooded house. She could not stand up. She had not eaten in five days. Katya said, We have to take her home.

I said, What? And watch her bleed to death? She's suffering, sweetie.

Katya said, It's not time.

Katya wanted to wait, and I talked her out of it. I'm not sure why. I think I believed Winona would suffer more. I hope I did not think about the burden she would place on me. The fact of my hope, however, proves I must have.

When the vet came back in, Winona did not swat him away. Her eyes were locked on mine. Katya was holding her head. My hand was on her neck. She did not fight when the vet slid the IV needle into her back leg. She did not flinch when he pushed the plunger. She kept watching me, watching. I think she was saying, Why? I know that's what she was saying. In thirty seconds, she was gone.

■ ■ ■

Katya was right and I was wrong. Winona was not ready to leave us. We should have brought her home and let her fight. She wanted to fight, at least a little longer. She wanted to rest her head once more on Katya's ankle and again lick Lincoln's cheek. She wanted to die on a bed in her house. She wanted to die in a warm place filled with love.

I killed her too early. I know that now. I might have known that then.

I also know, even as it was happening, Winona was already forgiving me.

But Lincoln took longer. He walked in the door at three thirty and dropped his backpack on the floor. Katya and I were there to meet him. He said, I'm ready to take Winona her card. We told him, and he wailed. He wailed a sound I hope never again to hear. He said, You promised me we could go visit her when I got home from school. He dropped to his knees and opened his pack. He was sobbing so deeply he couldn't breathe. He pulled out a card and said, I made this for her. You promised I could give it to her today. The card read, Winona, I love you and I miss you. Please come home soon. He had drawn her face and surrounded it with hearts.

My son said, How could you do that? I didn't even get to tell her good-bye.

■ ■ ■

ime does not heal all wounds. Some pain becomes part of who you are.

Six months after Winona died, I went running an hour before dawn, and heard her nails clicking on the concrete beside me. At breakfast, I spied Katya turn to scoop half her eggs into Winona's bowl; she seemed surprised to find it no longer there. At night, every night, Lincoln would say, I miss Nonie, and I would sit on the floor outside his room, slumped against the wall, powerless to accomplish anything worthwhile, while my son cried himself to sleep.

We needed distance between our memories and ourselves. The three of us flew to Germany to visit Katya's family. Katya wanted to spend a few more nights in the apartment Irmi and Peter had bought in Bernau, a small town in Bavaria, two hours south of Munich by train. Now a widow, her mom was going to sell the place. It made perfect sense to Katya, and it broke her heart.

We hiked, drank beer, ate schnitzel, and drank more beer. We went to the places Peter loved and talked about why he loved them. Katya said, Do you remember that couple we saw at Shingle Creek? I did remember. On one of our favorite hikes, we saw a man and woman celebrating their thirty-fifth anniversary. They had honeymooned at the Shingle Creek campground and were back to hike up to the crossing. The trail at the beginning is rocky and steep. We passed them less than a quarter mile from the trailhead. They were breathing hard. They asked us how much farther and we told them about four miles. They shook their heads in dismay. It had seemed so easy and short when they had done it last. They gave up and returned to their car. Katya said, I'm glad Papa was never unable to do what he loved. He would have hated getting old. I put my arm around her and pulled her closer. She said, So maybe it was better this way. But knowing that is not helping me miss him any less.

Five days later I flew home for a hearing. Katya and Lincoln would join me in a week.

While I was thirty thousand feet over the Atlantic, my client died in prison. He committed suicide on death row. There would be no hearing. When I was first appointed to his case, I had persuaded him not to give up his appeals, assuring him he had a strong legal claim. A letter he sent arrived two days after he swallowed an overdose. He told me he was sorry.

I had unexpected time on my hands. I sat down to play poker but found myself instead looking at pictures of abandoned Dobermans. I thought to myself, What's the harm? My plan was to fill out the forms at the Doberman rescue sites without telling my wife or son. That way, if we ever decided to get a dog, I would have already taken care of the approval process.

The Doberman rescue people scrutinize potential pet owners more thoroughly than the McCain campaign vetted vice presidents. I filled out forms that ran on for more than ten pages. I had to list multiple references, and the rescue league called them all. They called my neighbors and my vet without telling me. The day before Katya and Lincoln returned, Cindi called. She said, You have passed the background check. Now I need to inspect your home and conduct an interview. Can I come by tomorrow afternoon?

I figured I could just tell Katya and Lincoln Cindi was someone I needed to talk to about work. I said, Sure, tomorrow is fine.

She said, Do you want a puppy or an adult?

I'm not sure.

Male or female?

I don't know.

She asked, How soon do you want a dog if you are approved?

I said, I'm not sure I want a dog at all.

Two hours after I picked up my family at the airport, Cindi rang our doorbell. She walked in with a ten-week-old blue male named Franklin. I was not expecting her to show up with a dog. Lincoln looked joyful for the first time since Winona had died.

The first thing the puppy did was pee on the floor. Cindi unhooked his leash, and he went charging across the slate floor like he was plugged in. His legs splayed like a cheap card table bearing too much weight, and he skidded into the piano leg. It was like watching Tom and Jerry. Lincoln was laughing and chasing him around the house. Cindi said, Can we check out the backyard?

Franklin tore around the perimeter like some demented dervish. I had not trained a dog in more than a decade. I was not ready for this. I kneeled down and called his name. He launched himself at my face and his snout landed flush in my left eye. Cindi, meanwhile, had finished inspecting the fence. She snapped Franklin's leash back on, told me the house had passed, and said, I'll be in touch.

Katya said, What was that about? I told her I had just intended to fill out the forms so when Lincoln was ready for a dog, I would have done the paperwork. She shook her head and smiled.

Lincoln said, Dada, can we please get Franklin? Please?

I looked at Katya. She said, Is his name really Franklin? I nodded. She said, It seems like karma. I shook my head no. Her eyes locked on mine, and she mouthed a single word. Yes.

I said to Lincoln, Do you promise you will help me take care of him?

He said, Yippee.

Cindi called the next day and asked whether we wanted to adopt Franklin. Lincoln and I went to pick him up. On the drive home Franklin dropped his giant head in Lincoln's lap and plopped his right arm across his shoulder. Lincoln said, Thank you, Dada.

That night, with Franklin asleep in Lincoln's room, and Katya's leg draped over mine, Winona came to visit. The hair on her legs had grown back and her belly was flat. She smiled a Doberman smile. She reared up on her hind legs and put her paws on my shoulders, the way we used to dance. Then she started talking to me, which is how I know it was a dream. She said, I miss you all terribly, but that's not why I'm here. I'm here to tell you not to blow it, because you are getting another chance.

She pressed her snout against my neck, and her presence felt as real to me as death. It doesn't matter whether she actually said it, or whether I just heard it, because either way, those eight syllables, those five words, are the most important thing I've learned, the single fact that more than any other separates us from them, the lucky from the un.

And so, just in case I had not heard her the first time, she looked into my eyes, and she said them again.

You are getting another chance.

■ ■ ■

AUTHOR'S NOTE AND ACKNOWLEDGMENTS

The stories in this book are true.

During Peter's illness I kept a journal. In the weeks after his death, as my way of mourning, I used that journal to write a narrative of his final months. That narrative has formed the basis for this book. I wish desperately he were alive to confirm my memory of our conversations and approve the words I put in his mouth. I am confident that if he were, he would. And I am grateful to my mother-in-law, Irmgard Glockner, for allowing me to share his wisdom and his struggle. Peter's struggle with melanoma and Winona's death from liver failure took substantially less time to unfold than the Waterman case did. Consequently, while I cover the entire history of Peter's and Winona's ordeals, for narrative reasons, I have compressed the Waterman case into a shorter timeline.

My reports of conversations for which I was not present are based on contemporaneous accounts from at least one of the individuals who were there. In my reports of conversations between Katya and myself, I might have attributed my words to her and hers to me. I remember what was said, but I sometimes don't remember which of us said it.

Although all the events I recount occurred as I have described, this is a memoir, not a volume of history. In order to protect some confidential communications and the privacy of certain individuals, I have altered names and some identifying details.

Katya is my first reader. When she read an early section about Peter and said, *That's Papa*, she inspired me to finish the book. I also benefited beyond measure from the willingness of Mark Dow, Meredith Duncan, Dave Kajganich, Benjamin Musher, Lydia Musher, and Ron Turner to read the manuscript. Their wisdom as readers is exceeded only by their loyalty as friends. Additional thanks to my cousin Benjamin, one of the finest doctors I know, who spent quite some time with me discussing cancer treatment and etiology and saved me from many errors. Others who saved me from factual mistakes include Frieda Dow, Mark Dow, Karol Musher, and Laura Wittner. The mistakes that remain are attributable to either my obstinacy or my obtuseness.

For nearly a decade now, I have relied on my agent, Simon Lipskar, for much more than representation. His insight and counsel are what every writer hopes for. Cary Goldstein acquired this book when he was still at Twelve, and continued to help shape it even after he left. I am indebted to him, and to the entire team at Twelve, including Deb Futter, Sean Desmond, Brian McLendon, Libby Burton, and Tony Forde.

I am able to do the work I do because former Dean Ray Nimmer, Acting Dean Richard Alderman, and Associate Dean Lonny Hoffman have consistently supported the Texas Innocence Network and the death penalty clinic I run at the Law Center. And as I hope this book makes clear, the work itself is performed by a brilliant and tenacious team that I am proud to be a part of; the real names of the others on that team are Jeff Newberry, Cassandra Jeu, Erin Osborn, Kelly Hickman, Rindy Fox, and dozens of students and interns. They deserve far more than they earn, and they remind me every day that there are some people for whom improving the world we live in is its own remuneration.

ABOUT THE AUTHOR

David R. Dow is the Cullen Professor of Law at the University of Houston Law Center and the Rorschach Visiting Professor of History at Rice University. Nominated for a National Book Critics Circle Award for *The Autobiography of an Execution*, he is also the founder and director of the Texas Innocence Network and has represented more than one hundred death row inmates in their state and federal appeals. He lives with his wife Katya, their son Lincoln, and their dog Franklin in Houston, Texas, and Park City, Utah.